EBURY PRE...

THE DETOX DIET

Shonali Sabherwal is India's first practising macrobiotic nutritionist and chef from the Kushi Institute (USA). She started her training under Mona Schwartz, one of the pioneers of the macrobiotic diet. Her tryst with macrobiotics began in 1998, when her father was diagnosed with cancer, and she wanted to help him with an alternative approach to recovery. The mantle of being a 'cancer-curing' diet was given to macrobiotics in the mid-1970s, as it helped people recover and stay in remission from the most aggressive cancers.

Shonali started her macrobiotic meal business in 2008 and has previously written two books: *The Beauty Diet* and *The Love Diet*. She has a flourishing counselling practice and applies her core skills as a health practitioner. She has worked with ailments (over a thousand different cases) and helped reverse or keep them in remission. In 2020, she spoke to wellness experts on a podcast organized by Amazon Audible named *Soulfood Conversations*. She also won the Best Nutritionist award at Vogue Beauty Festival 2020.

She works out of Mumbai, conducts workshops across the country and has clients based all over the world. Within Bollywood, her clientele includes Katrina Kaif, Zoya Akhtar, Sidharth Malhotra, Hema Malini, Javed Akhtar, Esha Deol and Jacqueline Fernandez.

Contact:
Phone: 9819035604
Website: www.soulfoodshonali.com
On social media:
Facebook:
https://www.facebook.com/ShonaliSabherwalSoulFood
Twitter: Sh_oulfood
Instagram: Soulfoodshonali

ALSO BY THE SAME AUTHOR

The Beauty Diet
The Love Diet

PRAISE FOR *THE DETOX DIET*

'I have been following Shonali's recommendations for the past four months. Her passion for her work, her knowledge and the way she applies the principles to cleanse you and keep you balanced are fantastic. She covers the whole gamut of health foods suited for your condition and objectives, their incorporation in your diet and the recipes for you to follow. I feel great and have achieved what I wanted. The book is a step-by-step approach to health and well-being—highly recommended for everyone'—Sidharth Malhotra, actor

'If you tend to get stressed and find your body manifesting that stress in ways you can't explain, you need this book. We need to maintain our bodies, cleanse and fine-tune them. This diet does just that. It jump-started my vitality and it's a diet I'll keep going back to'—Zoya Akhtar, screenwriter and director

'Shonali Sabherwal is a revolutionary new-age health coach whose excellent personally crafted programmes will cater to your particular lifestyle and needs. Her care and encouragement will completely change your relationship with food. She has the secret formula for losing weight and keeping it off'—Sumeet Chopra, photographer

The
Detox
Diet

SHONALI SABHERWAL

EBURY
PRESS

An imprint of Penguin Random House

EBURY PRESS

USA | Canada | UK | Ireland | Australia
New Zealand | India | South Africa | China

Ebury Press is part of the Penguin Random House group of companies
whose addresses can be found at global.penguinrandomhouse.com

Published by Penguin Random House India Pvt. Ltd
4th Floor, Capital Tower 1, MG Road,
Gurugram 122 002, Haryana, India

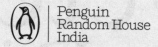

Penguin
Random House
India

First published in Ebury Press by Penguin Random House India 2017

ISBN 9788184007831

Typeset in Sabon by Manipal Digital Systems, Manipal
Printed at Replika Press Pvt. Ltd, India

www.penguin.co.in

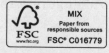

'The Earth is not just our environment.
We are the Earth and the Earth is us.
We have always been one with the Earth.'
—Thich Nhat Hanh

This book is dedicated to Dr K.G. Raveendran and
Dr P.T. Keshavan Nambisan
of Arya Vaidya Chikitsalayam,
two legends in the field of Ayurveda

CONTENTS

PART TWO

PART THREE

PART FOUR

FOREWORD

With lifestyle diseases growing at such an alarming rate in India, like autoimmune conditions, irritable bowel disease, diabetes, allergies, depression, food insensitivities, etc., Shonali's insight into how gut microbes are responsible for practically all health ailments is revolutionary. Today, research supports theories on strengthening the human microbiome (namely gut bacteria), and this has become a widely talked about subject in health circles all over the world. It lends itself to understanding what we truly need to optimize our health quotient.

We need health practitioners who understand what causes an imbalance in the human body. We also need food to be used as a tool to reverse these ailments. I have known Shonali for eight and a half years now, and eaten the food and done the detoxes she recommends to know how she uses foods to reverse health ailments, keep your weight stable, help your skin glow and make you look great.

I have always wondered what her secret is to setting everything right for her clients; now I realize that it is keeping the gut clean by maintaining a healthy balance amongst the colonies of bacteria and controlling inflammation. By doing what she does with the use of fermented foods, she helps us properly digest our foods and assimilate the nutrients from it.

Her detox approach is unique. I have always felt my skin glow, look more radiant and younger after I finished her detox diet. She already knew a major health secret before it even became a trend. This is what I admire about her—an immense knowledge of her field, her passion in using foods to help you, and remaining true to her work.

Forget dieting and start living, enjoying the food you eat. Do something that will create lasting changes in your life. When it comes to looking good, give your body the right inputs via foods. This will determine how you age—it's a lifetime investment.

Shonali has brought about a new way of thinking in this book based on scientific facts, and outlined a recovery plan that makes perfect sense. This book is an essential in your collection of health books. I recommend it to everyone looking for answers to longevity, good health and ageing. You will feel absolutely rejuvenated with the information she has brought out and the light she has shed on gut biodiversity being the key to your health.

INTRODUCTION

Isn't life one big detox? You should detox every day—not only from bad food but also from thoughts, bad relationships, negative emotions and unpleasant situations. If life could be one big detox every single day, you'd be one happy person. But that's where we usually go wrong. We keep things pent up—be they negative emotions, feelings, thoughts or even all the junk we eat. We let it fester inside us, till it finds its release in mental patterns that cause us harm or physical ailments that debilitate us. So the art of letting go is something one has to learn. That's where detox comes in.

This book is special and very close to my heart after *The Beauty Diet* and *The Love Diet*. It's my third child. Most children in this position find themselves in a 'zone of discomfort' with their parents. But like all mothers, I would like to nurture it, like I did my first child. Why? Because when it comes to being healthy, while my first book laid the foundation of creating a good blood structure, it's this book that will set the ball rolling on enabling you to live the best life you've ever had and for vitality 24/7. Knowing what you are on the inside results in the outward manifestations of health, beauty, abundant energy, mental clarity, strength, happiness and gratitude.

My Story: One Big Detox

I remember my friend Anu telling me, 'Gogi (my nickname), you are always on a diet!' While there is truth in this statement, I would say I've been on a detox diet every minute of every day for the last twenty-odd years. To achieve this, I have done two things that have laid the foundation of my life. First, I learnt how to practise meditation daily so that I don't carry any negativity, be it from situations or people. This ensures that there is no negative mental residue that might build up from my environment. Second, I have stayed true to a macrobiotic lifestyle for the last twenty-odd years, which makes for healthier blood, and is one true to the master detox lifestyle.

But I did not start here. I remember running out of the bathroom when I was ten, screaming to my mum that my period had started. When my mum checked, it wasn't my period; I was bleeding from my butt. I was officially declared to have got piles at the age of ten. While I know you all are thinking, 'Gory story! Why do we need to know this?' I'm narrating it because most parents avoid these situations when faced with it and don't know how to address them. The kid will then have to face issues in his/her adult years and that's what happened to me. The doctor told my mum to give me more milk—'*Isko doodh pilao* (give her more milk),' and never addressed my diet. My mum listened to the doctor. She tried to provide healthy Indian fare for us and was keen that we be vegetarian, like her. But my dad insisted on keeping us non-vegetarian, so there were a lot of animal products of all kinds on the table (always, even for breakfast) as well as loads of sugar, white carbohydrates and dairy. Little did I know that my stomach problem was the start of a bigger issue I was going to face years later. I was highly constipated as a kid and also developed back-pain issues (which everyone played down as having been inherited from my father) by the age of fifteen, so much so that I had to sleep on the floor most of the time. This was all interconnected: too much congestion in the stomach will eventually put pressure on the lower back.

I remember I was trying so hard to lose excess weight when I was twenty that I decided to visit all the dieticians in Mumbai. I tried one that recommended eating every two hours and drinking as much Diet Coke as I wanted. Another recommended eating cheese with every meal to increase protein intake and to eat up to seven eggs a day. One dietician said that it was okay to eat white bread or biscuits as long as my calories were kept down. I saw one who allowed white rice and sugar, again as long as the portions were limited and I ate every two hours.

Now that I look back, no one really addressed the deeper underlying issue—of a gut that was in poor shape, with the ability to absorb very little, and a build-up of bad microbes and an unhealthy ecosystem, which ultimately led to candida. None of the dieticians mentioned that the very foods they were recommending were actually feeding the candida. (The word 'candida' comes from a fungus called *Candida albicans*, which is one type of bad microbes; there are many different strains of good, neutral and bad microorganisms. It is the overgrowth of this fungus that leads to Candida-Related Complex [CRC] or candidiasis, also referred to as auto-brewery syndrome [ABS]).

It lives off sugar, dairy and a diet that most of us Indians have that is low in minerals. So in a sense we feed the bad microbes in our system almost on a daily basis, without being aware of it, with trigger foods, as I call them. Antibiotics and daily medication like blood pressure pills, cholesterol drugs and blood thinners only make their growth gather momentum in our bodies. While the so-called fungus (*Candida albicans*) lives within one's digestive tract and usually in woman's vaginas as well, it can spread itself throughout your body, like a carpet, on almost all organs and empty pathways—around your sinuses, wrapping itself around the spinal cord and nerves, and also accumulating at the base of the brain. It can also affect your organs: the heart, the lungs, the uterus (one of the causes for endometriosis in women), the liver—pretty much everywhere. It thrives on minerals, proteins and fats from your system, and leads to a depletion of minerals vital for your needs, like iron, selenium, magnesium, chromium, zinc, etc. This throws off the body's pH (a numeric scale to identify alkalinity and acidic nature of the body's fluid structure) and makes you the acidic. Now, the toxic waste that it throws out circulates throughout your body like a poison and weakens the immune system, which includes the endocrine (governing hormones) system as well. So people with this condition suffer from chronic fatigue syndrome, as it depletes the minerals that are required for both the thyroid and adrenal function. It has been linked to many common and autoimmune ailments: food insensitivities, allergies, migraine, fuzzy thinking, all digestive issues, colitis, vaginitis, loss of libido, low energy; and it is a precursor to thyroid malfunction, PCOD (polycystic ovary disorder), fibromyalgia, rheumatoid arthritis and cancers. While I had the overgrowth of one type of the so-called bad bacteria (*Candida albicans*), there are many such strains in the gut.

The diet methods applied by everyone I met were effective, but not in all cases. No one diet fits all, but that was the common approach they all adopted. None of them mentioned that they were actually recommending foods that would feed the bad bacteria and make them thrive, grow and never leave my body. No matter which diet I tried, I never lost weight or regained my bowel health.

I carried my gut issues into my teens and early twenties. By the age of twenty-six, I had started showing signs of constant thrush infections, the origin of which could again be traced back to my gut. But no doctor was pointing me in the right direction. My homeopath said it was psychosomatic, and the gynaecologist gave me topical applications like creams, suppositories, etc. No one addressed the diet and no one said it was due to something that lay deep in my system. I suffered for about five to seven years. I kept oscillating between the homeopath and the gynaecologist. I did start taking care of my diet a wee bit more, but was still doing everything wrong for lack of sound advice on all fronts. I was on all those foods that fed the candida, multiplied it and kept it trapped inside. Meanwhile, my back pain continued to haunt me, and finally, I was diagnosed with a slipped disc by the time I was thirty. I was bedridden for three months and walked around with a back brace. I was bloated, had constant indigestion, felt mentally fuzzy all the time, was not shedding weight and had terrible backaches and headaches. It was then that I sought the help of Ayurveda physicians from Kerala (details given at the end of the book) who told me that the root cause of all my problems lay in my gut.

While I was undergoing my first Ayurvedic *panchkarma* cleanse, I also joined the macrobiotic programme to train as a nutritionist/chef under the guidance of my teacher and counsellor, Lucci Baranda. She treated me inside out, instead of just focusing on the outside (i.e., calories and weight). She made me quit a lot of the main staples (white rice, dairy, sugar, refined flour and meats) which were harming me—they were pro-inflammatory (inflammation explained later)—and put me on a detox plan, restricting foods that triggered my insulin and spiked my blood sugar and fat-forming insulin (since insulin is a fat-building and fat-storing hormone, I was producing more insulin than required with poor dietary habits and had an overgrowth of the bad microbes in my system). Her approach was to starve the candida and cleanse my system off it. But she also did something else: she infused my body with healthy microorganisms via food (prebiotics and probiotics in layman's terms) that made me bounce back. While it took two years, I shed 10kg and looked like another person. I was on this plan for two years and managed to knock candida out of my system completely. For me, it was like knocking out cancer. Something that stayed with you since you were a kid gets worse as time rolls along, and one symptom bleeds into the other. It took twenty-five years of living with this issue, suffering all the time and my body's immune system breaking down for me to finally heal myself and prevent myself from getting into an autoimmune state in my later years. I did it with food alone. The entire world's population are living with varying degrees of imbalance that stem from the gut. We just don't know it. We also look at many of our health issues in isolation, as modern medicine looks at symptoms and treats a patient. We don't connect the dots to something that lies deeper, something that precedes the symptoms. Our problem starts in the gut—the engine where everything happens and where the combustion of all the fuel that you put into the body takes place.

In retrospect, my problems started when I was born; my mum suffered from candida (she has pretty much all her life). When she delivered me, the microbiota she passed on to me, if any, were not exactly healthy. We get our first set of microbes from our mothers when delivered vaginally. My mother had a normal delivery and so these microbes made up my gut ecosystem from the beginning. The saving grace was that I was breastfed for twelve months, so some substantial nutrition was passed on. Breast milk contains human milk oligosaccharides, or HMOs (which are also prebiotic), the main job of which is to nourish the good bacteria (the little that are there). The microbiota at this time has the ability to digest and extract energy from these HMOs. Hence, my mom was feeding my microbiome. These are the little bugs that eventually prepared me for solid foods. This is why you see infant formula marketers adding probiotic bacteria to their products, as they cannot mimic what HMOs do for the infant. I also remember that in my teen years, I took a lot of pain medication for headaches, period aches and the like. Brufen was a dear friend, subsequently killing all good bacteria and keeping the bad ones trapped in my gut. Plus there was my diet. Hailing from a regular Punjabi household, meat, chicken, eggs, milk, yogurt, paneer, sweets, white carbohydrates (simple sugars) and chocolates, and in my twenties, wine, beer, malts, etc., were staples—they all fed the candida. My own case history revealed itself to me once I started training to be a macrobiotic nutritionist/counsellor.

Another effect of candidiasis is the poisoning by acetaldehyde and ethanol, both of which are its toxic byproducts. Being poisoned by these two compounds is similar to having a hangover, as the ethanol (ethyl alcohol) levels in blood become similar to an alcoholic's. This is why it's called 'auto-brewery syndrome'. Your digestive system cannot handle sugar when it processes grain or carbohydrates of any sort, and could react to even moderately low carbohydrate foods like vegetables. It becomes like a brewery. It leads to the dilation of blood vessels, giving you headaches, palpitations and anxiety (I suffered from these symptoms many times); causes liver damage; and makes glutathione, an antioxidant needed by the body, inactive, aiding free radical damage (explained later) in the cells, accelerating ageing and initiating cancers.

Besides taking some twenty-five-odd years to knock it out of my system, it also led to various other issues— migraines, thrush infections, constipation, weight gain, puffiness, anxiety and, eventually, a weak back and slipped disc.

I would like to mention here that even the phase wherein you wean the child and introduce solid foods in the diet is extremely important in promoting the diversity of microbes within the child's gut. We should expose kids to a host of foods that will promote good bacteria (microbial diversity) in their guts. If you follow the principles of a high-fibre diet outlined in this book, adopt a plant-based approach (primarily), avoiding antibiotics as far as possible and introducing good fermentation (explained later in detail), it should be enough to create a healthy ecosystem for children. Just remember that you only have the first seven years of your child's life to lay the foundation.

My Background

I am a graduate in the macrobiotic approach to health, a qualified nutritionist, teacher and chef. Macrobiotics is rooted in the traditional Chinese medicine (TCM) system. I am trained in the art of the oriental system of diagnosis, which basically makes me qualified to read the health of your organs on your face (Chinese face-mapping) and also test for imbalances in your meridian lines—those that run through your organs. I use this system as a framework to arrive at a diagnosis and then a prognosis. I only use food to help reverse health ailments. However, I do bring in bodywork therapy (craniosacral therapy, acupuncture or acupressure), Ayurveda and homeopathy as well. I can safely say I am a food scientist or a food doctor. I know the healing properties of different food groups, and foods within those food groups, to reverse an ailment you may have. I try and work from the root of my clients' issues, reversing ailments systematically. My practice has led me to believe that almost everything stems from the gut. Whatever happens here governs the outward manifestations of the inside, i.e., the skin, hair, nails and also the way you look. The old adage 'You are what you eat' means just that and so much more. I think of it as: 'You reflect how clean your gut is.'

I use the Eastern medicine framework to treat my clients. An ailment for me is a state of imbalance in the body, and I simply use my tools (food) to restore the balance. Modern medicine looks at you symptomatically by compartmentalizing you. If your digestion is off, they don't look at it as being the result of your complete mental, emotional and physical make-up. They don't see that being a part of a complete body system, other things may be causing the indigestion. Instead, they prescribe a drug (which actually worsens your condition) that suppresses your symptoms for some time, only to crop up again later, and more fiercely. Using TCM as a framework, a person trained in the art of the oriental system of diagnosis looks at organs. Each organ is seen as a complex energetic system encompassing not only its anatomical entity, but also as being correlated to particular foods, emotions, tissues, sense organs, mental faculties, colours, climate, tastes, smells and more. The chart on the next page outlines these connections.

	EACH ORGAN AND ITS CORRESPONDING ATTRIBUTES						
ORGAN	TASTES	SOUND	COLOUR	EMOTION (NEGATIVE)	EXTERNAL ORGANS	BODY PARTS
KIDNEYS	SALTY	GROANING	BLACK	FEAR	HAIR	UNDER EYES
LIVER	SOUR	SHOUTING	GREEN	ANGER	NAILS	BETWEEN EYEBROWS/ EYES
SPLEEN/ PANCREAS	SWEET	SINGING	YELLOW	ANXIETY/ PENSIVENESS	LIPS	LIPS/ TEMPLES
LUNGS	PUNGENT	CRYING	WHITE	GRIEF/ DEPRESSION	BODY HAIR	CHEEKS
HEART	BITTER	LAUGHING	RED	SAD	COMPLEXION	NOSE (TIP)

HOW TO READ THIS BOOK

At the outset, I would like to define two terms that are crucial to this book and used throughout. The word 'gut' refers to the gastrointestinal tract, comprising the alimentary canal, i.e., a tube-like passage that begins at the mouth and ends at the anus. This is where digestion, absorption and elimination of leftover (unabsorbed) food take place. Also, when I refer to the microbiota/microbes/microorganisms in the gut, I am referring to those that form a part of the digestive system, i.e., those mainly in your intestines, because this is where the largest and most important microbial community in the body resides. It plays an important role in your overall health.

So basically, microbes = microbiota = bad and good bacteria = microorganisms.

The book will give you action plans to follow a detox on two levels: (1) if you want to just do a mini-detox, i.e., if you want to restore the balance of your system after coming back from a vacation, want to look great for an event or just want to step up your health; (2) if your digestive system gives you regular trouble, and you want to retune the whole body to restore the balance by cleansing, taking you to the next step of your health.

Part One lays down the theory on which the whole system of cleansing or detoxing is based. It outlines why we need to have a good inner ecosystem, i.e., a strong healthy gut (as explained earlier), with its own microflora and microfauna (bacteria). It seeks to make you aware of the origins of microbiota (bacteria), which we direly need, what causes its breakdown and what ends up giving us a leaky gut. It simplifies the workings of an organ that often remains unexplored. This part is essential to the understanding of what makes your gut strong and what finally causes inflammation and ailments and what reflects in outward expressions of energy, vitality and health.

Part Two puts into practice the basic tenets of a detox. It takes you through the various phases of a detox and why they are so important. So it would be a good idea to read each phase and let it percolate for a bit before moving on. Each phase has its own plan and its own dietary recommendations, so please read the entire section before starting any one phase.

Part Three sets the different detox diets in motion—the raw juice detox, the regeneration detox and the master detox diet. This part will need careful reading. You may choose one detox over the other, depending on the results you are looking for.

The book in a nutshell does the following for you:

(1) Highlights what causes ageing, stomach or gut-related problems, autoimmune ailments, weight gain and poor health.

(2) Tells you how to bring about changes on a deeper level in the body by improving gut (stomach) health.

(3) Reveals secrets of the ultimate anti-ageing and antioxidant-rich detox plan.

PART ONE

1

YOUR FORGOTTEN ORGAN

You Are Not 'You', but Microbiome

I remember my teacher S.N. Goenka saying in one of his discourses (on ego) as part of a ten-day vipassana course that if you were to turn yourself inside out, you would be one mass of cells talking to another mass of cells. He later went on to explain that we are just that—a mass of cells, and that we are actually born without any ego. This is something we create when we develop attachment to our so-called 'self'.

We are born pure, unfettered and uncontaminated. But did you know that the moment you exit the birth canal, you start picking up the microbes from your environment? As Raphael Kellman says in *The Microbiome Diet*, 'You become 90 per cent microbe.'[1] If we look at ourselves, we are 10 per cent human and 90 per cent microbes. The collection of microorganisms that make our bodies their home are called human microbiota, and microbiome (the genetic code of each microorganism) is a miniature world of non-human organisms (microbiota) that flourish within your gastrointestinal tract. When you look at this world inside us, our ego (as Goenka-ji says) is simply a figment of our own imagination. This attachment to the 'I', 'me' and 'my' falls flat.

Another thing explained again by Goenka was the theory of how we humans have all the elements of the universal energy around us within us: we are made up of tiny *kalapa*s (atoms), and each kalapa has the earth, water, air and fire element, like that around us, with its microorganisms. In the same vein, we are the earth, with the same elements: all the trace minerals and oxygen, hydrogen, carbon combined. We are changing every day with great speed, i.e., new kalapas are generated every minute, the old ones are dying and they interact with great force. This change within the body is the same as the pattern followed by microorganisms: new ones come in, old ones die.

The different communities that reside within us are like different sects or cultures living in different parts of our bodies. For example, the bacteria living in your digestive tract are different from the ones that live in your lungs. It's almost as though we exist as ecosystems and not as individuals. For the purpose of this book, we will focus on bacteria as well as the yeasts, viruses and parasites that make up your gut microbes. These are the body's microbiota that help you fight against disease. Despite being healthy, you carry these microbes in your hair, skin, between your teeth, under your nails and inside you. You have more bacterial cells than human cells, so you can only imagine the quantum of microbes.

So far, we have managed to be right about the food we can see with the naked eye, i.e., plants, animals and fungi. But those that can be seen only under a microscope have been neglected. It is only now that we are looking beyond 'bad bacteria'.

Think of your gut as a garden—rich and green. Go ahead and visualize it. Now think of these friendly microorganisms inhabiting that garden. How you choose to build the soil (i.e., the nutrition through food) to keep these microorganisms nourished and healthy is entirely up to you. This is the key to everything in your life. This plays a crucial role in our health and outward manifestations of it (skin, hair, nails, glow, weight, attitude and a whole lot more). According to me, this is the missing link in all diets.

Everybody has a different set of microbes depending on how they were born, the varying food they eat, people they interact with and the environment they grow up in. Not even 10 per cent of your microbes may be the same as the people living with you. This is what precisely accounts for you being predisposed to certain aliments while others may suffer from a completely different set of ailments (or not have any). The character of your microbiome can change depending on your diet, how many sexual partners you have, whether you have pets or whether you are firstborn, second-born, etc. Your microbes define what it means to be you.

The microorganisms that live within you dictate the way the food is used in the body: they control cravings, govern appetite, influence genes and your hormones, make natural antibiotics, produce vitamins needed to survive, aid sleep, control your moods by controlling your neurotransmitters, and act as a detoxification unit (like a second liver) in your intestine. For example, your gut microbes help you break down complex carbohydrates. Your body wouldn't be able to do this on its own. The same microbes reduce the toxic build-up in your liver from the unhealthy food you've eaten and help with elimination. When they find outsiders or substances that are not native to the gut, they guard you against them.

The bottom line is that these microbes live everywhere, in and on your body. If you look at the microbes by weight alone, according to Rob Knight,[2] an adult carries three pounds of microbes. This makes your microbiome one of the largest organs in the body, equal to the weight of your brain and a little lighter than your liver. Each microbe is different from the other; the ones that exist on our skin protect us from other dangerous outsiders that might try to infect us. Yet, different parts of the skin will have differing microbes. For example, women tend to have more diverse microbial communities on their hands than men do. The ones in our nose and lungs are different from the ones in our mouth and stomach. The ones in our mouth also help regulate blood pressure by releasing nitric oxide which helps relax our arteries. Our gut has its own immune system, and some microbes send signals to control inflammation and also establish whether you will get an autoimmune disorder. There are many vitamins you would not make if it were not for these microbes. They help produce short-chain fatty acids (SCFA), which protect you against cancer, besides helping with inflammation. Setting the foundation for the right microbes starts early in life, and if we neglect this (as in my case and maybe in yours as well), it sets the tone for inflammation, candidiasis, leaky gut syndrome, weight gain and other diseases in the future.

If you look at your intestines—it is a thirty-foot long sewage system, housing the largest community of microbes in the human body; a warm and cosy environment with no shortage of food and water. So while the small intestine is where all the nutrients from the food are absorbed, it is the large intestine where water is absorbed. It is also where fibre is fermented by the microbes that live here, which passes undigested from the small intestine. The microbes here are considered to be the gatekeepers of our metabolism.

So it comes down to this: The secret to fast and permanent weight loss and revving up your metabolism and energy levels, having beautiful hair and skin, reversing ailments and balancing your mood swings is the microbiome—the trillions of tiny bacteria that live in your intestines. An imbalance will work against the diet. Just balancing it will make you get the results you want. I promise you will have this knowledge once you get to the end of this book.

Microbiota: A Brief History

In the nineteenth century, Louis Pasteur experimented with microorganisms and discovered that they caused food spoilage and fermentation. Pasteur's study of beetroot fermentation quickly convinced him that fermentation was a biological process. His first study on the subject, *Memoire sur la fermentation appelee lactique,* was published in April

1857. He wrote, 'Fermentation is a correlative of life and of the production of globules, rather than of their death or putrefaction.'[3] Pasteur spent his life as a crusader, studying microorganisms. He led the way for a new way of thinking about the happenings in the environment, their effect on foods and the process of preserving them. His discoveries paved the way for many who later came out with fermented foods.

In the 1960s, Abigail Salyers began studying bacteria from the human gut. She focussed on one such species called bacteroides, long before studies revealed that these bacteria are connected to human health in multiple respects. Justin and Erica Sonnenberg in their book *The Good Gut* describe her as being a fearless microbiota pioneer and a pragmatic experimentalist.[4] They visited her lab, which had all the hallways filled with artefacts from her microbiota experiments. She revealed that bacteroides could survive oxygen exposure (whereas most other gut microbes wither when outside of the oxygen-free environment of the gut). She said this species were adept at consuming dietary fibre. She and her contemporaries laid the foundation of understanding how many bacterial species subsist in the gut—by eating portions of plants that we as humans cannot digest on our own.

In the 1980s, another project called the Human Genome Project took centre stage. This study aimed at sequencing all the genes of the human genome. It took thirteen years and one billion dollars to complete it. The importance of this project, however, was that it pointed researchers in the direction of understanding diseases better. In their book, the Sonnenbergs[5] conclude that there is sufficient research done in this area to now make diet and lifestyle adjustments to optimize the health of microbiota, and thus our overall health. They say, 'By understanding how we first acquire our microbiota, how and what it eats, how it taps into our immune system as well as every other aspect of our biology, and what happens to it after a round of antibiotics, we can make informed choices that maximize the health and resiliency of this most important community of hitchhikers.'[6]

How We Get Our Microbiome

As I mentioned earlier, the first set of microbes come from your mother (so the way she has eaten all her life is crucial). During pregnancy, specific kinds of lactobacillus dominate a woman's vagina. The microbe strains from her gut draw out extra energy from foods, and this manifests in her vagina as well. Research is still to confirm if the uterus has microbes that are passed on to the foetus; however, it does point to the placenta and amniotic fluid having microbes. Technically, she gives you the first set of microbes, for your gut as well, providing the foundation for things to come. This does not hold true for C-section births, since the microbes are picked up from the mother's vagina during birth. A baby born via a C-section will only have microbes picked up from the mother's skin and those she may come in contact with post-birth. The microbes we have when we are born keep changing; once we are adults, we have a different set and many more strains of microbes than when we were young. The antibiotics and vaccinations we are given as babies literally kill colonies of these microbes, but we build these up quite rapidly within a few weeks. Our diets are the key to shaping the character of the ecosystems in our bodies very early in life. For example, a baby who is breastfed has a different, healthier set of microbes than a baby who is formula-fed. This is because certain sugars in breast milk promote beneficial bacteria. These microbes change character when we are fed solids. What we eat over a period of time keeps altering the microbes in our bodies. Another thing that affects children in their early years is the environment. As Rob Knight explains: Kids put their fingers in their mouth after sticking them into everything. Siblings, pets in the house, living on a farm or visiting one exposes the kid to a varied number of cultures of microbes. The more diverse the set, the healthier kids will be.[7]

In short, the people you interact with, your hygiene levels, things you touch, pets and everything you come into contact with play a part in this.

We have moved from being agrarian to leading more urban lives, therefore our contact with the environment is at abysmally low levels. As explained earlier, 90 per cent of our bodies are made up of microbes living inside or as they do in the environment around us. Hence, there is a need to establish practices (daily lifestyle inclusions) that bring back microbes and bacterial strains into our guts. We come into contact with microbes daily—through the ones that live in us, the ones that 'check in' and check out' daily and the ones that we get from the 'earth', by which I mean our contact with dirt or soil. The ones that check in and check out also come to us via a handshake or close contact with someone, or through the food we eat. We reduce our microbial diversity in a super clean environment and further reduce it with the trigger foods (the foods that deplete the good microbes or increase the bad ones) we include on a daily basis. That's why the presence of a pet increases the microbial diversity in you and your kids. A study quoted in the book *Eat Dirt*[8] by Josh Axe that appeared in the medical journal *Clinical and Experimental Allergy* showed that having pets may improve immune system and reduce allergies in children. As many as 566 children, who had pets, including cats and dogs, were studied, with blood samples taken from them when they turned eighteen. They found that children who had cats exhibited a 48 per cent decrease in allergies and those with dogs exhibited a 50 per cent decrease in allergies. The explanation given was that kids are exposed daily to the pets that play in dirt, making this a great way to get some of that interaction with dirt or soil. These micro-exposures add up over time and help the good microbes in your gut, ultimately boosting immunity. Antibiotics are another cause for a further decline in microbial diversity.

Examination of Gut Microflora

The great Spanish painter Salvador Dali would record details about his motions daily. His *Diary of a Genius* is a book before its time, rightly voicing concerns about gut microbiota. His elaborate description of his stool each day supports this view of his: 'I increasingly dislike all scatological jokes and all forms of frivolity on the subject. Indeed I am dumbfounded at how little philosophical and metaphysical importance the human mind has attached to the vital subject of excrement.'

In Ayurveda, the basic indicator of all diseases is said to be abnormal excrements. In an ancient manuscript *Bhrigu Samhita,* there is a description of microbes (kitanus) in the intestines. It states: 'There are kitanus in each and everybody. But when some toxic gas (*dushita vayu*) or *dravya* affects these germs adversely, the number of pathogenic germs reaches the climax. The person in such a situation is said to suffer from infection (*krimi-roga*). The disease is characterized by the spread of millions of germs in the wall of the intestines. When the germs inhabit the abdomen, they do not allow the proper digestion of food, causing diarrhoea, fever and other disorders, leading to dysbiosis, a condition of microbial imbalance in the digestive tract. In a nutshell, dysbiosis occurs when the inner ecosystem is in a state of imbalance, quite simply explained, when the bad microbiota outnumbers the good ones.'

2

LEAKY GUT AND INFLAMMATION

Are You Suffering from a Leaky Gut?

According to a paper by Hari Sharma,[1] in the Ayurvedic system, dysbiosis can produce *ama*, a toxic state that initiates and promotes disease-related processes throughout the body. The optimum functioning of the gastrointestinal (GI) tract requires proper mucosal integrity and balanced microflora. If these two aspects are out of balance, it produces ama. The body views ama as a foreign substance, and reacts by producing antibodies, giving rise to antigen–antibody complexes and resulting in immune disorders. Hence, it blocks channels and leads to the spread of disease. The accumulation of ama at various places in the body varies from one person to the other and causes different afflictions. For example, if it gathers at the joints, it can lead to arthritis; at the blood vessel level it is seen as the accumulation of lipids, which cause plaque formation and reduce blood flow. At the cellular level, damage can occur at various sites. Damage to cell receptors can hinder the action of hormones and other biochemicals at the cell level, and damage to the DNA can cause mutation and the initiation of cancer cells. Ama can also deposit in the liver and harm it. A healthy cell structure in the GI tract, including proper functioning of the villi (small projections that protrude from the epithelial lining of the small intestine's walls) and tight cell junctions (the spaces between epithelial cells that are sealed tight and allow only fully digested material to be absorbed) are important for the intestinal barrier. The human intestine, while absorbing nutrients from the food we eat, also functions as a barrier that prevents harmful pathogens (microbes) from entering our body or bloodstream. If someone has a 'leaky gut', it means the tight junctions are compromised due to increased use of antibiotics, exposure to bad bacteria and/or certain trigger foods. The toxic stuff which actually should be eliminated will then seep through the walls of the intestine into our bloodstream. This leads to an immune system breakdown, if not corrected. This then increases the toxic burden, which leads to inflammation and disease.

The causes of leaky gut are inflammatory bowel disease (IBD), Crohn's disease, NSAIDs (non-steroidal anti-inflammatory drugs or painkillers), altered flora in the gut, small intestine bacterial overgrowth (SIBO), coeliac disease (resistance to gluten), infection, food allergies, peptic ulcer disease, chronic alcoholism, diarrhoea, strenuous exercise, increasing age, nutritional depletion, poor dietary choices, stress and emotions, systemic disease, low stomach acid and exposure to toxins.

How do doctors in India test for leaky gut syndrome?

A good doctor will send you for:

(1) An IgG (immunoglobulin G) test, which checks for food allergies in the body.
(2) Rule out parasites, generally done via a stool test, also checking for a balance of good and bad microorganisms.
(3) A breath test called the Lactulose Breath Test or LBT (lactulose is a non-absorbable sugar), which is done to rule out SIBO and diagnose *Helicobacter pylori*. The test will diagnose the hydrogen and methane levels in the blood (not done in India).

Sharma's paper noted about 500 different species of gut flora (microbes/microbiota). The positive effects of these are salvaging energy from carbohydrates, synthesis of B and K vitamins, balancing pH, production of SCFAs (explained in detail later), stimulation of the immune system and production of anti-microbial compounds. Nearly 70 per cent of the human system's microbiota is localized in the digestive tract. An imbalance in the gut microflora, with an overgrowth of the bad ones as opposed to the good ones, will lead to dysbiosis. Causes of dysbiosis are attributed to impaired digestion, hypochlorhydria (basically low stomach acid, leading to undigested food remaining longer in the stomach than it should), overuse of antibiotics throughout one's life, presence of high levels of ethanol (ethyl alcohol) in the blood due to yeast overgrowth, overuse of pain-killers, decreased peristalsis (movement of food through the digestive tract), impaired immune status and dietary factors.

Is Your Digestive System on Fire?

One of my patients, Rashmi, thirty-two, a mother of two kids, found herself unenergetic, overweight and extremely stressed. She came to me after exhausting all her hope in allopathy medication. That's when people generally come to me, when their gut linings have already been destroyed by drugs and

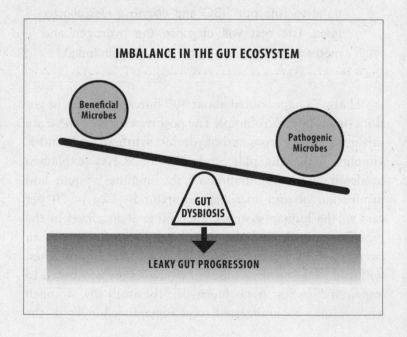

LEAKY GUT PROGRESSION & CONSEQUENCES

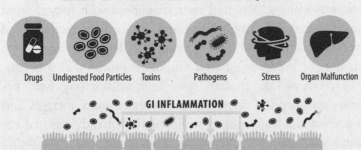

Drugs Undigested Food Particles Toxins Pathogens Stress Organ Malfunction

GI INFLAMMATION

IMMUNITY
AUTOIMMUNE DISEASE
FOOD SENSITIVITIES

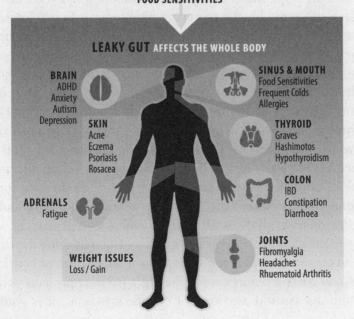

LEAKY GUT AFFECTS THE WHOLE BODY

BRAIN
ADHD
Anxiety
Autism
Depression

SKIN
Acne
Eczema
Psoriasis
Rosacea

ADRENALS
Fatigue

WEIGHT ISSUES
Loss / Gain

SINUS & MOUTH
Food Sensitivities
Frequent Colds
Allergies

THYROID
Graves
Hashimotos
Hypothyroidism

COLON
IBD
Constipation
Diarrhoea

JOINTS
Fibromyalgia
Headaches
Rhuematoid Arthritis

antibiotics. In her quest to get healthy, I was the sixth person she was visiting. She had been diagnosed with hypothyroid (or Hashimoto's thyroiditis) and was on medication and antidepressants. She had vitamin B12 deficiency and I also diagnosed her with adrenal fatigue. Rashmi's diet was fine, but it seemed as though something was wrong with her body's absorption. Her IgG test revealed food allergies and I suspected a leaky gut as well. She had already reached the full-blown stage of inflammation. I told Rashmi if she didn't fix her leaky gut, she would not be able to absorb anything that went into her body, from food to medication.

I started her on a programme of whole foods (foods that are considered good quality), fermentation, prebiotics and a diet rich in the fibres that good microbiota thrive on. I also gave her bone broths to repair her stomach lining (more on bone broths later). She said she was already managing her stress levels with yoga and meditation, and was under a good psychotherapist. After one month on the plan, she dropped 3kg and was sure she wanted to go ahead with it for at least the next three months as advised. In another three months, her vitamin B12 levels came back to normal (which was a sign her gut lining was on the mend for sure), her cortisol levels dropped, and the insulin as well as fasting blood sugar levels were stable. After staying on the plan for three more months, she lost 11kg. She was beaming and glowing from all the health benefits she was experiencing.

Our digestive system fits inside our bodies quite neatly and compactly, but if you were to lay it out in front of you, it would cover a tennis court. The digestive tract protects you from disease and any kind of outside infections; it is your immune barrier—your gatekeeper. It works extra hard not only to extract nutrients from your food but also to sort through and deal with the stockpile of undigested food, new microorganisms and the ones already present. This gang of microorganisms are a mix of good guys, bad guys and the ones that are neutral. I can't emphasize enough that the more diverse your gut microbes, the healthier you are. They protect you from harmful pathogens entering your gut, but only if the friendly ones outnumber the unfriendly ones. However, when this does not happen, you reach a state of dysbiosis. Over a period of time, dysbiosis will then lead to leaky gut syndrome. The overgrowth of bad microorganisms can cause your intestinal lining—which is slightly permeable and allows only nutrients and water to seep through the barrier of the gut—to become more porous, allowing toxins to escape directly into the bloodstream and cause a host of issues. In his book *Eat Dirt*, Josh Axe refers to a study by Alessio Fasano at the University of Maryland who brought out of the closet the protein zonulin, which causes the tight junctions of the gut wall to loosen. The three things that trigger the production of zonulin are exposure to bacteria, increased antibiotic use and exposure to gluten.[2]

Another patient, Arun, came to me with fibromyalgia, an autoimmune condition characterized by chronic pain throughout the musculature and tissue in the body, and fatigue. He also mentioned he was suffering from IBD, which was a condition he suffered from before he was diagnosed with fibromyalgia. He had tried everything and had found no respite. He ran his own business, and his stress levels were extremely high, though that is common to most of us today. He was managing his condition with physiotherapy but felt that he had to resolve his IBD first. He was right of course.

His food habits revealed a lack of good fibre in his diet and too much of refined white flour—pasta, cereal, bread, biscuits, crackers. He was also on a lot of pain medication, and had a habit of not chewing his food thoroughly. His blood tests revealed low levels of vitamin B, including B12, vitamin D and zinc. Also, a diagnosis done by me revealed there was an overgrowth of pathogenic yeast and depletion of certain good probiotic strains. I gave him a protocol I follow with my IBD clients—a diet high in digestive enzymes (probiotic-rich foods), prebiotic foods, grains (minimal at the start, as he was reacting to sugars), vegetables and good cold-pressed oils (fats). I also removed all trigger foods that fed his condition and the yeast overgrowth. In a month he found himself springing with energy and in three months he reported an 85 per cent reduction in pain. Arun is not the first IBD client with an autoimmune condition I have worked with. I have seen many with different permutations and combinations of ailments, but the precursor is always IBD, followed by the autoimmune condition.

What Is Inflammation?

If I told you to close your eyes and think of inflammation, what comes to your mind? This is what my mind will conjure: redness, swelling, rawness, pain and infection. Even if you thought of two of the aspects I listed, we are on the same page. Inflammation is the body's coping mechanism to outside elements that it cannot assimilate or recognize on the inside. Now imagine all that I told you happening to someone's body over time. It turns into systemic inflammation. Modern medicine has not started recognizing the correlation between systemic inflammation and disease. You could have varying degrees of inflammation, and in many ways, the macrobiotic diet, by controlling certain factors—i.e., bringing in the balance of yin and yang—helps keep the body's inflammatory response under check.

Everyone remembers studying about white blood cells in school. I remember my teacher saying they are our soldiers who are supposed to ward off external elements in the body. Our body is constantly protecting us, and for this, our white blood cells need to be fortified well. When it loses the ability to realize what needs to be done to protect the body, its response is to go into an autoimmune condition. This phrase is used often these days, especially with reference to your thyroid disorders. Therefore, inflammation and immunity are interlinked. Chronic inflammation will eventually lead to a weakened immunity. Like the lady who walks the rope in a circus and does a perfect balancing act, our body attempts to achieve that perfect balance between inflammation and strong immunity. A key factor in this whole act (think of the stick that this lady holds to balance herself) is the microbes in your gut. If you were exposed to the right ones and have ones with the right characteristics, the balancing act is easy. But if your gut houses more of the bad variety, you are definitely a prime candidate for inflammation. Some microbes release toxins inside the body (endotoxins, which are toxins within bacteria). One particular kind is called lipopolysaccharide (LPS), which eventually leads to systemic inflammation. The body reacts by sending cytokines (powerful immune messengers that fire several other cells) into action. This sets the inflammatory process in motion, like a gigantic snowball rolling down a hill, gathering speed and trampling everything that comes in its way. Dr David Perlmutter in his book *Brain Maker*[3] talks about LPS, a combination of lipids (fat) and sugars, and a major component of the outer membrane of the cells of certain bacteria known to tip the inflammatory pathways of the body. LPS-protected bacteria represent 50–60 per cent of the gut bacteria. Studies on MS (multiple sclerosis), Alzheimer's disease, inflammatory bowel disorders, diabetes, rheumatoid arthritis, depression, lupus and autism have all indicated elevated LPS markers in patients suffering from these ailments. Similarly, in the case of a leaky gut too, LPS gets into the bloodstream.

The presence of LPS in the bloodstream is a huge precursor to all autoimmune conditions. All my clients who have an autoimmune disorder suffer from some kind of gut-related issue caused by their diets, stressful lifestyles and lack of knowledge about the right foods for this condition. Leaky gut syndrome leads to various ailments like asthma, autism, inflammatory bowel disease, skin issues such as eczema, psoriasis and urticaria, IBD, Crohn's disease, ulcerative colitis, diabetes (type I and II), multiple sclerosis, severe migraine, rheumatoid arthritis, fibromyalgia, thyroid, adrenal and chronic fatigue, lupus, NAFLD (non-alcoholic fatty liver disease), and of course, systemic inflammation that precedes cancer.

A lot of clients who come to me with insulin resistance are also overweight, and an analysis usually leads me to the fact that they have chronic inflammation in their gut as a result of bad bacteria. This is similar to the situation I was in.

Before I move on to how inflammation impacts you on several fronts, I'd like to explain one word that I will bring up constantly—'ecosystem' and its link to systemic inflammation. It is defined as a community of microorganisms interacting with each other. So, when we are going down the ski slope of our lives, we are gathering momentum and taking in everything that our environment is throwing at us food-wise. We are no longer mindful of what we put into our bodies. We are responsible for destroying this intricate balance of our ecosystem. A happy ecosystem of the gut achieves a delicate balance between the friendly and unfriendly bacteria. However, ingesting chemicals as a result of eating food that is not washed properly (that's why the stress on organic), having junk food, sugar, dairy, white refined flour (*maida*), popping medication and living under stress, strips us of everything on the immune system front, leading to systemic inflammation. It predisposes you to an autoimmune condition.

The Immune Barrier: Your Gut

Think of your immune system as the gatekeeper to your health. It protects you against external pathogens, parasites, viruses and most of all disease. Your immune system is further classified into the innate immune system and adaptive immune system. If you have a cut, bruise or injury, your innate immune system kicks in. The adaptive immune system has its own memory and remembers past injuries. When your system is attacked repeatedly by a host of bad microorganisms, your innate and adaptive immune systems have to keep changing gears, which overtaxes them. Now while fighting these invaders, antibodies (basically proteins created in response to driving harmful pathogens out) are created by the immune system. To protect you, the antibodies attack healthy cell tissue as well—creating a state of chaos within the body. Let's look at the biggest ailment facing us today—malfunction of the thyroid. Like a garbage truck that comes in to collect garbage, the antibodies clean up good and bad cell tissues of the thyroid, causing the body to switch to an autoimmune state. Hence, prolonged imbalance of microbes in the gut eventually leads to an autoimmune state.

'Our gut microbes communicate constantly with the part of the immune system located in the intestine.' These 'conversations', as Justin and Erica Sonnenberg call them in their book *The Good Gut*,[4] help our body discriminate between harmless entities like food or havoc-creating microorganisms like salmonella. It is the microbiota that helps train the immune system to make the distinction. Our immune system is highly mobile. Immune cells living in the intestine and 'conversing' with the gut microbes can move to new sites anywhere in the body. A T-cell (one of the major classes of immune cells found in the body), which lives in your intestine today, may be in your lung or spinal fluid tomorrow. And that cell can remember its experiences with the microbes in the gut. Say, a particular T-cell encounters an invading pathogen while spending time in the intestine. It can multiply into many cells and spread throughout the body to inform other tissues of the impending danger. If that pathogen crops up in the lungs, the educated T-cells are ready to help fight that infection.

The microbes in our gut control the responsiveness of the entire immune system. They dictate the small processes of immune response like a fever, to a larger response like determining how long you will stay with a cold. A good microbiome is positively correlated with a strong immune system. An imbalance causes the T- and B-cells (also termed the killer immune cells) to attack harmless cells, triggering an autoimmune response.

Autoimmune conditions do not just come on suddenly; they creep up over time. It is my belief that acute stress over a prolonged period of time will eventually cause you to get there as well. The body will throw you signals, much ahead of you being hit with an autoimmune condition. Typically, these are: constant allergies, headaches, skin issues, asthma, dryness in throat or mouth, thyroid, pain in joints or tissues, IBD, chronic fatigue, thyroid (hypo or hyper) and constant urinary tract infections. There are many conditions associated with being autoimmune. Here are the most common ones known to us: rheumatoid arthritis, Graves' disease associated with hyperthyroidism, Hashimoto's disease associated with hypothyroidism, lupus, coeliac disease, multiple sclerosis, ankylosing spondylitis, type 1 diabetes, alopecia, Sjogren's syndrome, fibromyalgia, psoriasis, eczema, myasthenia gravis, chronic fatigue syndrome, inflammatory bowel disease and sarcoidosis.

In his book *The Microbiome Diet*, Kellman quotes a study done in 2004 by Dr Paresh Dandona,[5] wherein he asked his research subjects to consume two kinds of breakfast sandwiches: one made of egg, ham and cheese, and the other sausage on a muffin. He measured their blood levels for C-reactive protein (CRP), a marker used to test for inflammation. His subjects' rate of inflammation skyrocketed within minutes and remained high for hours. Eventually, he discovered that foods high in refined carbohydrates, processed sugar and unhealthy fats encourage the growth of certain types of gut bacteria. The bad bacteria overwhelm and drown out the good bacteria as soon as they get a taste of unhealthy fats and starch. The substance called endotoxin is produced, which pushes the system towards inflammation.

One of my patients, Arshiya, came to me with psoriasis. She had gone everywhere possible for a cure. First of course was the traditional route of allopathy. They gave her drugs and topical creams which suppressed the condition only temporarily. She never knew that her diet held the key to getting rid of her issue completely. She showed me her skin, which was in bad shape. She had the prettiest face, but she was ashamed of her patches.

She also complained of constipation, and a diagnosis revealed that she was depleted of the good microbes in her gut. She did have a leaky gut, which laid the foundation for a lifelong case of inflammation. It had led her to this autoimmune state of psoriasis.

I started her on a regimen for psoriasis, first avoiding lactose (milk and dairy products) and also making her stay away from wheat, sugar and refined flour. She came from a meat-eating family and had a penchant for chicken. I told her to stick to fish alone. It was difficult, but she wanted to give it a sincere try. With a diet rich in digestive enzymes, whole grains, vegetables, fruit, healthy fats from coconut oil, ghee, avocados, some superfoods and a supermom who cooked for her, keeping her challenged (a good caregiver always helps), her symptoms started abating in four months. There were no new eruptions, and the old patches started giving way to normal skin. She has been told to stay on this plan for two years. Now that she has a grip on the diet plan, she is determined to get rid of this condition.

Take this quiz to find out if your inner ecosystem is out of balance:

(1) Have you taken medication/antibiotics over a prolonged period at any time in your life?

Yes   No

(2) Do you have a tongue that is coated white, especially in the morning?

Yes   No

(3) Do you suffer from constipation or a loose stomach often?

Yes   No

(4) Do you consume a lot of milk and dairy products?

    Yes   No

(5) Do you consume a lot of sugar or sugary drinks?

    Yes   No

(6) Do you often suffer from fuzzy thinking or feel mentally spaced out?

    Yes   No

(7) Are you in a state of fatigue very often?

    Yes   No

(8) Do you suffer from bloating, indigestion or heartburn after eating?

    Yes   No

(9) Do you have an autoimmune condition like thyroid or any other?

    Yes   No

(10) Do you suffer from allergies often?

    Yes   No

(11) Do you fall sick very often (more than twice a year)?

    Yes   No

(12) Have you been diagnosed with IBD (ulcerative or Crohn's disease)?

Yes   No

(13) Do you get frequent migraine?

Yes   No

(14) Do you suffer from joint pain or tissue or muscle pain?

Yes   No

(15) If you are a woman: do you suffer from UTI (urinary tract infections) or thrush infections?

Yes   No

(16) Are you intolerant to many foods, e.g., wheat?

Yes   No

(17) Do you have a lot of stress which you find overwhelming?

Yes   No

(18) Do you suffer from swinging moods?

Yes   No

(19) Do you have any skin issues (e.g., spots, psoriasis, eczema, urticaria)?

Yes   No

(20) Do you suffer from bad breath?

    Yes   No

(21) Do you suffer from insomnia?

    Yes   No

(22) Do you have dry mouth or throat?

    Yes   No

(23) Do you crave bread and white carbohydrates?

    Yes   No

(24) Do you crave alcohol?

    Yes   No

(25) Have you taken birth control pills for more than two years?

    Yes   No

If you answered yes to more than five questions, you definitely have a case of bad microorganisms outdoing the good ones and need to alter your diet to create a healthy ecosystem. If you answered yes to more than two but less than five questions, you are beginning to build an unhealthy ecosystem.

A Trip through Your Digestion Process

One of the questions I ask my clients in every consult is, 'How are your bowel movements?' Some provide details, while others who want to indicate they are fine say, 'Oh, great', by which they usually mean they go once a day. Most people are reticent to talk about their digestion and bowel movements. 'Fine' and 'all right' don't sufficiently describe the intricate workings of the gut. Most people think if the food goes in and comes out, the digestive system is working fine. One of my friends, who has IBD, has a theory—anything he eats has to act like a plunger in his stomach, so he keeps running to the loo. In reality, he suffers from colitis—a condition that is not really helping with his immunity.

Healing your gut or preventing a leaky gut starts with knowing exactly how your food is digested. The bedrock of your digestive system is the GI tract. The digestive system encompasses your liver, gall bladder, pancreas, gut microbiome, nervous and circulatory system (which transports blood, nutrients, oxygen, carbon dioxide and hormones to and from cells).

Chew, Chew, Chew to Get Good Poo

Mary Roach in her book *Gulp: Adventures on the Alimentary Canal*[6] describes the digestive system as a highly elaborate inside of the tube that starts at the mouth and ends at the anus. Before we even get into what happens when a bolus (i.e., the food in your mouth) gets into this tube, let's address an important facet of pre-digestion: chewing—a much neglected lifestyle habit. At the Kushi Institute where I trained, we are told first to eat by ourselves in the dining hall, and chew each bite fifty-two times. When I entered the dining hall for the first time and saw an American girl chewing like a cow, I burst out laughing, only to be told by my friend Connie later that I eat way too fast. This in part explained my history of poor digestion and became another vital lesson in reversing my digestive sickness to health.

Roach compares the way you chew to the way you fold your shirt. She describes chewers to be fast, slow, long, short, right and left chewers. Some of us chew up and down, while others side to side. Your oral processing habits, she goes on to say, are a physiological fingerprint. The jaw is vigilant and knows its own strength. The faster and more recklessly you close your mouth without giving it a conscious thought, the less force the muscles are willing to apply. She further describes in her book that the 'oral device' comprising teeth, lips, tongue and saliva work together to form a bolus—a mass of chewed, saliva-moistened food particles or a 'swallowable-state'.

Two interesting things happen while chewing, both related to the enzymes in our body. Firstly, ptyalin, which is required for the digestion of carbohydrates, is released in saliva. The other thing is that the brain kicks into action at this point, recognizing whether you are chewing protein, carbohydrates or fat and accordingly tells the stomach to secrete the right enzymes, e.g., pepsin in the case of protein.

Once the food is in your stomach, the cells in the stomach lining release hormones, including digestive enzymes, to keep the whole process of digestion going. Acted upon by various enzymes, the food is converted to a semi-fluid liquid called chyme. The hydrochloric acid helps break down the protein and release digestive enzymes to aid digestion. If your stomach is low on this acid, you will end up getting acid reflux and small intestinal bacterial overgrowth (SIBO), which will eventually lead to a leaky gut. From the stomach, the chime is whisked away to the small intestine, wherein proteins, fats, vitamins and minerals are extracted with the help of enzymes produced by the gall bladder, liver and pancreas. More than 80 per cent of the nutrients are absorbed here. In case certain fats are not digested, more bile might be required. As Indian diets are usually heavy in fats (refined oils), this is usually the case for Indians. Bile is produced in the gall bladder and this is why a person who has had gall bladder removal surgery is at a high risk of developing a leaky gut. After the chime reaches your colon (large intestine), what remains is mostly fibre, the food for your gut microbes to feed on. Here two key processes take place: (1) fermentation of the fibre—done by these microbiota or bacteria in your gut; (2) production of SCFAs, which in turn help the colon by promoting good cell growth, increasing absorption of water and providing a barrier to diseases that stem primarily from the gut. Don't confuse SCFAs with fats (oils). SCFAs are chains of carbon and hydrogen, an acid group at one end of the molecule. Their job in the body is to either provide energy or form the structure of cells. SCFAs also contain butyric acid or butyrate, which is found in ghee (that's why we Indians advocate ghee so much). Butyrate is known to have positive effects on insulin sensitivity, intestinal permeability, maintaining gut barrier integrity, increasing absorption of water in the gut and hence preventing leaky gut syndrome. If fats and fibre are properly balanced, with the right proteins and low-glycaemic foods (which don't overload the body with sugar), you get the right balance of SCFAs. These molecules are also known to stimulate the fat-burning activity of the microbes and help the intestine gather up T-regulatory cells (a type of immune system cell), which the body produces after an immune response. A scarcity of these will lead to autoimmune conditions, IBD and, in some cases, cancer. Your gut microbial diversity drives SCFAs in your gut, which in turn affects the processes of your gut.

One indication of having bad bacteria or microbiota is that you react to almost any fibre. The one thing you need to digest it is good microbiota. One of the hallmarks of macrobiotic approach is the use of fibre derived from complex carbohydrates, namely, brown rice, millets, vegetables, legumes and nuts. Most weight loss enthusiasts think that carbohydrates make them fat. Where they go wrong is in failing to distinguish the type of carb. Your inner ecosystem needs this fibre to build diversity, otherwise it breaks down. The key is to achieve the right balance—not too many, and yet not too few. Therefore, it is always important to remember that the type of food you eat is more important than the number of calories you consume. How many calories your gut bacteria are actually extracting for you is a fact that is unknown; the right approach is to eat good-quality fibre, healthy fats, high-quality protein and the right carbohydrates from whole grains. For example, those who have studied the Hazda (hunter–gatherers in Africa) say they consume 100–500g of fibre per day.[7] The Hazda microbiota houses a much greater diversity of microbes than a Western one or for that matter, an Indian one. An average Indian consumes about 28g a day[8] from 215g of carbohydrates.

The Stomach Acid Connection

Your stomach acid—the excess or lack of it—can create a host of issues affecting gut diversity. It makes food more digestible, but can also kill microbes. Saliva is the first place where bad bacteria are sifted out of your system. Similarly, the stomach acid (namely, hydrochloric acid) is the second place where microbes are killed. Therefore, maintaining the balance of your stomach acid is crucial to preventing the growth of unhealthy bacteria. Stomach acid tends to decrease when your health is compromised or you are under stress. Acid reflux occurs when there is not enough acid. This causes food to remain undigested, making it unable to pass on to the small intestine. This is when the stomach acid is pushed back up your oesophagus and you notice a burning sensation.

What Do Gut Microbes Do?

If we are doing well on the microbial diversity in our guts, the assumption is that 85 per cent are good or neutral bacteria and 15 per cent are the bad guys. The good ones prevent the bad ones from making a home in our gut. The intestinal lining which is protected by cells acts as a barrier, working to sort out the good and bad microbes, and protect the gut. Consider it to be the gate of a castle (your digestive system). The entry points of your gate (the junctions of the intestinal lining) allow the good guys to enter and 'frisk' the bad guys, checking if they can be let in. When the gate weakens due to large amounts of poor microbiota, the bad ones start entering, causing dysbiosis and eventually leading to a leaky gut.

Good Gut Bite

Garlic has shown to be very effective in treatment against bad pathogens (bacteria) due to its antifungal properties. To activate these properties, it needs to be chopped or crushed. This forms an antibacterial chemical called allicin, which gives it its antifungal nature. Ajoene is another compound which ascribes the same to garlic.

Contraindication: Advisable to get a physician to okay its use if you are on blood-clotting medication or if you are of *pitta* condition (according to the Ayurvedic tradition).

3

YOUR MICROBES AND DISEASE

Now that we understand how the microbiome can cause systemic inflammation over a period of time, let's examine how it impacts different parts of you and how it is revealed as different kinds of ailments.

Weight Gain

Remember my story? No matter what diet I went on, I was not able to shed my excess weight. I stuck to every principle espoused: eating every two hours, consuming high-protein foods like eggs and cheese, etc. Nothing worked. I exercised like a fiend, but that did not work either, till the connection was made years later. My gut microbes had a huge role to play, and the food I was eating was a colossal trigger to making them multiply. After correcting just this one aspect of myself, I shed 10kg. Thus, I maintain that gut microbes had more to do with my weight loss than anything else.

Manjeet Hirani, a commander flying for Air India, came to me with an issue of stomach bloating, puffiness, acidity and excess weight. She said nothing ever worked. A pilot by profession, she said she indulged in coffee, sweets and other stuff that came with a hectic lifestyle. However, she also had a sense that dairy was the trigger for her problems. I found that she was harbouring unhealthy gut bacteria and had candida. I put her on the detox approach—we eliminated the list of foods to avoid and introduced a wholesome, natural approach by adding a lot of rich bacteria through food, which you will learn about in this book. She felt amazing when her weight dropped and the puffiness came down. Most of all, she no longer craved unhealthy foods and felt a surge in energy. This came as a result of a raised metabolism. Here is what she had to say:

'I had a severe stomach issue. My stomach had become as hard as a stone. I was totally bloated, constipated and had a severe burning sensation. I went to several doctors and they gave me antibiotics. One of them even gave me sleeping pills saying it's due to stress. One day I read an article by Shonali in *Mumbai Mirror* about gluten intolerance and how it can play havoc with the system. I figured out I was lactose intolerant and wanted to explore how foods were triggering my condition.

'I immediately contacted Shonali, who took my whole case history. She said that I had too much of bad bacteria in my gut and had to be supplied with good bacteria. She diagnosed me with candida and put me on her candida-control diet plan. She put me completely off wheat, milk, milk products, sugar and yeast products. I was introduced to the wonderful world of good digestive enzymes through the miso in my dahls and soups, and quick pickles. In my subsequent visits to allopathic doctors, I was detected with *Helicobacter pylori* bacteria. The doctors suggested a treatment with antibiotics and prescribed a diet plan which Shonali had suggested in advance. However, the doctor's don't tell you that the antibiotics itself destroy the stomach. I not only knocked off weight, but was well again in four months. Thanks to Shonali, who was bang on. I visit her whenever I have a gut issue.'

Gut microbes control your appetite, cravings, metabolism, decide how calories are extracted from food, and how to utilize them and where. It is important to eat food that restores our inner ecology, keeps us balanced, satiated and gives us a strong microbiome which can ward off anything. In this state of balance, we can lose body fat quite easily.

Not all bacteria are bad. Here is one piece of good news on why *Helicobacter pylori* can actually be helpful for you.

Helicobacter Pylori Has Just Got a 'Bad Rep'

You may have heard of *Helicobacter pylori*, which has housed itself in our stomach for so long as the cause of ulcers or other stomach-related ailments. Hence, most people who have it think of it as something really bad. However, it also has benefits—not only does it regulate the acid production in the stomach but also ghrelin—the hormone that tells your body when it is hungry. It also regulates leptin, another hormone. When the microbiome is balanced, leptin rises as ghrelin falls, signalling fullness after a meal and giving you energy. If you do not have *Helicobacter pylori*, then you will have difficulty in shutting off the hunger signal.

As we have established that what you eat alters your microbiome, making it more hospitable for certain strains of microbes and less for others, let's look at specific examples. People who eat meat may have very different strains compared to those who eat a lot of carbohydrates. In his book, Rob Knight highlights a study[1] wherein Peter Turnbaugh, a systems biologist at Harvard University, and his colleagues got some volunteers to either go on a vegan diet or have a diet of red meat and cheese. Veganism caused little immediate change to their gut microbes. But the meat-and-cheese diet caused considerable changes overnight, increasing the kinds of bacteria linked to cardiovascular disease. Hence, a bad diet can have an almost immediate consequence on one's microbiome.

So stop counting calories, stop cutting back the carbs and stop avoiding oils or fats. It is a known fact that weight loss is deeply related to irregular blood sugar levels, whether your fat is burned or stored or how hungry or full you feel. The hormones in the digestive system are also important in this song and dance of weight loss. The more stable they are, the more likely you are to lose weight. Raphael Kellman, in his book *The Microbiome Diet*,[2] demonstrates this point with a study. In March 2013, three groups of mice were tested with the following criteria applied to them before being put into groups. The first group went through a fake surgery, to ensure that surgical trauma was not a factor that predisposed them to weight gain. After the surgery, they were given unlimited fatty and sweet foods to eat, and they gained weight. The second group was given a calorie-restricted diet, and they of course lost weight. The third group actually went through the gastric bypass surgery, and were allowed to eat as much as they liked, and they lost weight too. The calorie-restricted (dieting) group and the gastric bypass group showed some differences. The dieting mice continued to suffer from high insulin and glucose levels. If your insulin and blood sugar levels are high, your body is doomed to fail on a diet. The mice that had the surgery had normal insulin and glucose levels, despite being given unlimited access to food, and kept their weight off. Researchers concluded that the surgery had reset the mice's hormones and altered the microbiome of the mice. However, this does not mean that gastric bypass surgery is the way to go. This is just to draw your attention to the fact that altering your gut microbiome can help you achieve weight loss as opposed to restricting calories. A natural precursor to getting obese is an unhealthy ecosystem; a gastric bypass surgery addresses this issue by changing the gut microbiome. However, I am suggesting natural ways to achieve it in this book.

Hormones are crucial in determining how blood sugar levels are processed within your body, how fat is stored or burned and how satiated you feel. When they are out of order in your digestive system, you tend to eat more and convert food to fat, hence gaining weight. So, the number-of-calories-consumed theory falls flat here. A further experiment on the same mice also proved how the microbiome plays a key role in weight loss. From each of the three groups of mice, microbiota was transplanted to another three separate groups of germ-free mice that had no microbiome of their own. The germ-free mice implanted with the microbiota from the gastric bypass microbiome group lost weight, even though they had had no surgery. They just needed the microbiome of the mice that had the surgery to lose weight. An important regulator in the lipid metabolism, again governed by the gut microbiota, is angiopoietin-like protein 4 (ANGPTL 4), also known as fasting-induced adipose factor (FIAF), which helps metabolize the triglycerides that gets deposited in your fatty tissue. A weak microbiota will have less of it in your body, and more triglycerides stored in the body as fat.

Obesity has been linked to an inflammatory response in the body. Recently, an actress considered heavy went through a three-week regimen at a Western wellness spa, and came back looking sexy and slim. It was like she had had a complete makeover, and it was the talk of the Bollywood fraternity. Then, another who had been to the same place for entirely different goals also came back completely changed. Before they went, they were in chronic states of inflammation. One due to the dairy, sugar and fructose consumption and the other because of gluten intolerance. What the wellness spa had essentially done was to control their inflammation, thereby impacting their weight. Obesity is associated with pro-inflammatory cytokines which come from the adipose (i.e., fatty) tissue itself. These cells cause disruptions in the functioning of the human system from within as well. The visceral fat that exists around your belly and organs produce inflammatory molecules that load up the liver. In all inflammatory conditions, fat-generated cytokines are always elevated.

My weight has remained stable for the last ten years, even though I put in 'x' number of calories (mind you, I don't count as I believe in the quality of calories and not the number attached to it). I work out, I would say, pretty intensely. Therefore, enough expenditure takes place as well. So my body weight remains the same, due to something that I am doing right. In fact yours should too, if you are a healthy individual. Several studies point to the fact that when you go into a calorie deprivation mode, the body will hang on to more fat. This explains why yo-yo dieters regain weight once off a diet. When you are in this mode, the body will keep you from gaining weight because you expend more calories and consume less. However, this is only till you get off the diet plan and regain all of it. The body has, as Gerard Mullin says, a 'set point',[3] which remains constant, maintaining your body weight in a stable range despite minor changes in calories. The body will also hold on to weight when deprived of calories. That's because the body's set point has shifted downward and is telling your body that your metabolism needs to be slowed to minimize weight loss during periods of caloric deprivation. This gives you an insight into how low-calorie diets have a short-term efficacy as the new set point limits weight loss. Overall, it is harder to lose weight than gain weight. Yo-yoing weight loss is a common result of weight loss programmes, and causes you to ultimately weigh more. It raises the body's set point, which means the brain tells your body to increase body weight to reach this new equilibrium and sends control signals, so that you gain weight and fat mass. Thus it becomes harder to lose weight as the set point is raised each time a weight loss regimen fails. When I was at Kushi Institute, I was amazed to see people fill up their plates with all kinds of wholesome natural foods. I kept thinking of the calories they were consuming. Of course, this was when I had just started my training as a nutritionist/chef in the macrobiotic approach. What was also amazing was to see how healthy and slim they were; they were glowing. I too did the same for the four years that I went back and forth to my institute. I ate that way in a controlled setting. Back home, I practised the same on myself. Poof! Two years later, I was another person.

Any dietician/nutritionist will tell you that the lead-up to gaining weight has a lot to do with you being insulin-resistant, leptin-resistant and having visceral fat (fat around your organs, mainly the belly). However, no one will point out how inflammation feeds into all of these factors; most go by the calorie-in-and-calorie-out model of losing weight. This actually puts you in a trap for later, making the body's set point harder for losing weight. For one, toxins, released when in a systemic inflammation condition, block insulin receptors, making it difficult to convert calories to energy, but easy to store fat. Leptin, the hormone that keeps you satiated, is also interfered with. Fat invites more fat, so the area around your organs, specifically the belly starting under the ribcage, pretty much covering all your organs and going right down to your pubic bone, except the lungs, is where you put on maximum weight (sounds familiar?).

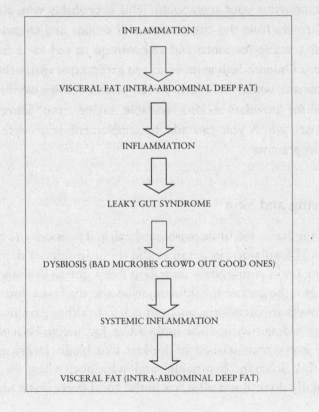

INFLAMMATION

VISCERAL FAT (INTRA-ABDOMINAL DEEP FAT)

INFLAMMATION

LEAKY GUT SYNDROME

DYSBIOSIS (BAD MICROBES CROWD OUT GOOD ONES)

SYSTEMIC INFLAMMATION

VISCERAL FAT (INTRA-ABDOMINAL DEEP FAT)

> ### Good Gut Bite
>
> Inulin, found in all the prebiotic food suggested in this book, is something of a wonder among plant fibres. It has the ability to absorb excess glucose in the system and improve the metabolism of fats. It also helps you digest food and make you feel full. This fibre, which your microbiota love, helps them produce some key vitamins supporting your metabolism. This is probably why our farmers have the cheap option of onions and chapatti as a staple for lunch and still manage to toil for a full day. Onion is high in inulin, as are garlic, asparagus, *leekh*, banana, wheat and chicory root (used in coffee blends). Inulin powder is also available online (see Source List), which you can add to supplement your detox programme.

Ageing and Skin

Ageing has a lot to do with gut health. The more the free-radical (explained in detail in the top-it-up phase) damage going on in your system on a daily basis due to dysbiosis in the gut, the greater the inflammation and the faster you age. Humans are often vain, and as much as health is paramount, every woman wished she looked like Jacqueline Fernandez and every man wished he looked like Hugh Jackman or Hrithik Roshan. Justifiable, and why not, when we can actually do it. But it all starts in the gut. I don't know about their guts—but the outward expression is exactly a mirror of what you are on the inside. The largest organ covering your outsides is your skin (glow or clearness), followed by hair and nails. A breakdown on the inside will, of course, affect the outside.

If you read the latest research on age and cancer, ageing is marked by a multiple decline in the body's cells and tissues. When cells experience oncogenic stress (i.e., stress that might cause cancer), cells go into cellular senescence,[4] wherein there is irreversible growth of the cell. Inside each cell, our genes are arranged along twisted molecules of DNA called chromosomes. At the end of chromosomes are stretches of DNA called telomeres, which protect our genetic data; they hold the secrets to how we age and get cancer. They have been compared to plastic tips on shoelaces, because they keep our chromosome ends from fraying and sticking to each other, which would destroy our genetic information. If cells divide, the telomeres get shorter and when cells can no longer divide, they become senescent or inactive. This is when ageing begins and cancers could arise. Inflammation accelerates the shortening process of the telomere and this can be reversed with the right foods, right lifestyle, introduction of the right power foods and antioxidants.

Glowing skin—isn't that what everyone wants? I get a facial done once in three months. The reason I do it is that Anjali (of The Ageless Clinic, Oshiwara, Mumbai—thanks to Dr Harshna Bijlani) gives the best facial massages. It allows me to just zone out. It gives me those forty-five minutes of deep sleep. She keeps trying to convince me to try her age-lock packages, but I tell her that no matter how much she tries, I simply don't believe that one can achieve long-lasting healthy skin by using a machine or through treatments. I'm sure Dr Bijlani will disagree. But I believe that a lot of what your skin says is reflective of how your gut is doing. It is dependent on the microbial diversity you have, which translates into your blood condition and that reflects on your skin.

Your skin has a direct correlation with your gut microbes. Inflammation and a weak gut will always impact the skin directly as these microbes are responsible for extracting nutrients needed by the skin from the food you eat. For example, beta-carotene found in red peppers and all coloured vegetables converts to vitamin A, which is used to repair and renew skin. Trace minerals like copper and zinc help build collagen, and selenium protects it from free radical damage (explained later). Less absorption of these minerals also causes hydrochloric acid to go down, which in any case declines with age. At the same time, vitamin B7 (biotin) is made by the microbes of your gut—much needed for hair, skin and nails. Vitamin B12 is something you get from the gut of animals. Most vegetarians, especially vegans, have deficiencies in this vitamin, and the only place where it can exist is where fermentation takes place, i.e., where good microbes exist. We get this from good-quality fermented products (outlined later in greater detail). Vitamin B12 is responsible for carrying oxygenated blood around, so it is necessary for glowing skin and producing vitamin K. This is something that a healthy microbiome does easily, while a compromised one doesn't do at all, or does marginally. Our guts are lined with a host of these friendly microorganisms that protect us from taking in toxins released by unhealthy foods that do not assimilate and the environment.

My former client and friend Ritu always had excessive sebum, a wax-like substance. When the body is in balance, the sebaceous glands produce a healthy amount of it to lubricate the skin. However, when the body's pH is thrown off, an excessive amount of it causes the pores to get blocked and is one of the causes of acne. Tired of her chronic problem, Ritu said, 'Shonali, what do I do? No matter what I eat, this sebum does not go away.' I knew the key was to work on her diet, making sure it was rich in enzymes. She could have tried creams and gone for many age-lock treatments. She also had dark bags under her eyes. According to the oriental art of diagnosis, which I practise, her kidneys were definitely depleted and there was a lot of adrenal fatigue. The kidneys hold on to fear as an emotion, which Ritu later revealed she had ever since she stepped into the adult world. First it was the fear of her parents, then her husband and in-laws. It took her two years, with continued effort and commitment from her end, to resolve all her issues.

We needed to improve the condition of her blood and get her acidosis (a condition in which the blood is more acidic and less alkaline) under control. Eating whole grains, vegetables, legumes, fruit and leafy greens, along with a lot of fermentation and supplementation via superfoods eventually led her to the path of complete recovery. She worked on her emotional issues alongside. Being on a cleansing approach helps clear up negative emotional energy as well.

Dr Nigma Talib, in her book *Reverse the Signs of Ageing*, talks about the concept of 'digest-ageing'—how gut microbes affect the ageing process.[5] Malabsorption and mal-digestion don't allow your skin to thrive. Poor collagen renewal and the hardening of elastin fibres lead to lines and wrinkles, and increased inflammation in the skin. This, in turn, accelerates ageing, causes acne, rosacea (wherein facial blood vessels become enlarged, giving the skin a reddish look, almost like a rash), dark circles and poor circulation, which ends up impacting skin glow. If you want younger-looking skin, you must look after the bacteria that populate your gut.

Elaborating on the concept of 'digest-ageing', she says that not only does absorption of nutrients affect the skin but also, when gut bacteria are not healthy, inflammatory substances released by bacteria destroy our skin and fatty acids that actually protect our skin against inflammation. Low levels of lipids (which hydrate the skin) cause dryness and puffiness under the eyes. Instead of protection, there will be rapid damage and wrinkles as the skin comes into contact with UV(ultraviolet) rays and pollution.

We've all heard that proteins are the building blocks of our skin. When protein is broken down into amino acids, the cells choose what they need to build new tissue. This is extremely important for skin renewal. It is the one source of food groups to repair dead cells. Muscles, hair, skin, eyes, nails and cells make up your organs—lungs, liver, heart, kidneys, sex glands, nerves and brain—all need protein. Once food hits the small intestine, the pancreas kicks into gear with lipase, which breaks up fat; amylase, which handles carbohydrates; and protease, which breaks down protein. It is extremely important to keep the supply of enzymes active at all times, on all fronts, as each food group needs them to help synthesize and extract nutrients. Some vitamins are fat-soluble while the rest are water-soluble, which means you need fat to transport them and break them down; if this process is affected, they pass out of this big tube.

Your Attractiveness Dimensions Rooted in the Organs, Nourished by Basic Approach to Foods

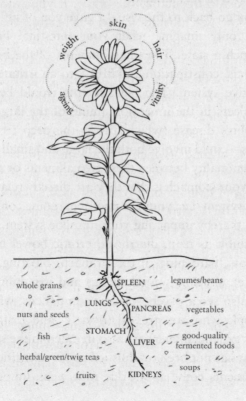

Irritable Bowel Disease

Simply put, IBD is the inflammation of the digestive tract. It affects your gut, which is not only the seat of everything but also an important organ vis-a-vis inflammation. I think most people suffer from some degree of IBD. In my practice, the ratio of this ailment to others I treat is 70:30. The attack of an unhealthy set of microbes will first most likely impact your gut. Therefore, it's essential to understand the implications of this ailment.

If you go back to the visual I gave you of inflammation, you can only imagine what your intestinal lining looks like in such a state. The small ailments of the bowel range from colitis, constipation and SIBO, to an irritated intestine or digestive system. The big ailments would be ulcerative colitis (ulcers in the innermost lining of the large intestine) and Crohn's disease (which affects the deep tissues of the intestines—could involve both the large and small intestines). The commonality between these two ailments or anything to do with your stomach is that they are directly related to your inner ecosystem (i.e., your gut microbes) going completely out of order, thereby impacting your immune system. Symptoms could exhibit as pain, diarrhoea, erratic bowel movements, weight loss, hardening of the stomach, bloating, flatulence (excessive), anaemia, mood swings and irritability. In many cases, I also see a psychosomatic component, which means that people who are stressed (overtly) and irritated in the mind (as explained later) are also irritated in the stomach.

What has not been established so far scientifically is that these ailments come about due to a weak immune system or an imbalance of the inner ecosystem or a combination of both. In my opinion, it's the imbalance that impacts immunity. From my macrobiotic learning, it is clear that what you eat either nourishes your body or throws it off balance. So either you are providing good bacteria daily, staying clear of antibiotics and painkillers, and keeping the inner ecosystem thriving, or destroying it by eating crap. There could be some tendencies predisposing you to a condition. For example, someone who is gluten-intolerant and does not know it, but keeps eating it over time may also start destroying the lining of the gut.

Roweena came to me with a chronic IBD situation. I remember when she walked in she said, 'I am always fearful of stepping out of my house and have become antisocial as my condition does not allow me to be away from the toilet.' She was in a state of full-blown inflammation, and diagnosis revealed severe candidiasis. She also constantly suffered from urinary tract infections. She said she was pushed to a consult by her family and friends. She was not able to shed weight, but was more concerned about her current IBD condition.

I started her off on the programme with lots of good-quality fermentation (explained later; but mainly food that adds digestive enzymes to break down and absorb nutrients from your foods, giving you good probiotics) to nourish her with probiotics, and loads of prebiotic foods as part of every meal. I added lots of immunity strengtheners and supplements with alkalizing foods. Completely avoiding trigger foods and staying away from raw food (which in a compromised digestive system is difficult to digest), Roweena stayed super compliant. The therapy provided amazing results—she lost 5kg in four months, the inflammation was brought under control, the abdominal swelling disappeared, there was no UTIs and it was all happiness. Roweena has stuck to the programme and says she never thought she could feel this way. This is what she had to say:

'Shonali has been a boon to me. I was referred to her by a dear friend. I was apprehensive for a year, but one day decided to give her diet a try. It is something I have not regretted for even a single day. I have been suffering from IBD (or IBS), which indirectly gives me anxiety and affects my immune system. Shonali's way of treatment, through Indianizing the macrobiotic approach, using supplements and a simple diet (where I don't have to go about looking for my ingredients, etc.), has made me feel calmer, hence sorting my gut problem. Basically, she's brought about a balance in my mind and body through foods, giving me more energy and confidence. My advice: please don't look for immediate miracles. You do feel a bit taken aback when she stops you from adding sugar to your tea or coffee. But she's only stopping the killers. I am feeling 75 per cent better since I started her diet last August (2015); I have lost 5kg. I'm on the path to wellness.'

Dr Josh Axe, in *Eat Dirt*, classifies malfunctioning guts into five distinct kinds: candida gut—which is found in most people who are overweight and have yeast overgrowth; stressed gut—which is caused by stressed adrenals, thyroid and kidneys, causing hormonal imbalances, fatigue and thyroid disease; immune gut—which affects people with food allergies, inflammatory bowel disease and autoimmune conditions; gastric gut—which affects people with SIBO and acid reflux; and toxic gut—resulting in gall bladder, skin and chronic liver issues.[6]

Whichever kind of gut you have, the bottom line is keeping it rejuvenated with a host of friendly microorganisms and making sure the bad microbes stay away or drown out, such that a balance is maintained. As Mary Roach points out in her book *Gulp*,[7] some of the most beneficial polyphenols (now being touted as a beneficial antioxidant in coffee, tea, fruits and vegetables, known to fight cancer), which are micronutrients, cannot be absorbed in the small intestine without colonic bacteria of the good kind. The same holds true for charred red meat which has been termed as a carcinogen. However, it is the raw material for making carcinogens. With the right gut bacteria to break it down, the raw material is harmless. Thus, changing people's bacteria is turning out to be a more effective strategy for treating issues and prevention of disease than changing their diet.

Let's Talk Poop

In my macrobiotic training, we have three classes (nine hours) dedicated to the subject of poop or potty or *kaka*, as Indians call it. Most of us confuse quality with quantity. A 'big dump' always makes people happy. Many people I know walk out after a big dump and think they have conquered the world. But that's not right. In the words of my teacher John Kozinski,

- It should be long, like a banana (long sausage), S-shaped
- Not smelly
- Medium to brown colour
- Not like pebbles, but smooth
- Slide out gently
- Not fall like a big stone
- Not stick to the toilet bowl (indicative of mucous)
- You shouldn't push or strain; it should be done quickly (you can't be singing songs and reading the paper on the throne; that's not what kings or queens do)

Allergies and Asthma

Rob Knight, in his book, asks the reader to think of the immune system as a radio. If you're dialled into a specific station, you can hear the music crystal clear, but if you're in between stations, random signals come in the way and cause loud, unpleasant static. In a similar way, the immune system may find something to latch on to if there is no signal. If you're lucky, it can be the pollen or peanut butter that spikes through the static, causing allergies; if you're unlucky, the immune system might latch on to your own cells, causing diabetes, multiple sclerosis or other autoimmune diseases.[8]

As Dr Axe says in *Eat Dirt*, 'We don't just live on the Earth, the Earth lies in us.'[9] He means this quite literally. As

Expanded Bristol Stool Chart with Personality Typing

Type 1	Separate hard lumps, like nuts (hard to pass)	Perfectionistic and exacting, you hold high standards. Your ideals can be burdensome, but your meticulous work stands out in a crowd. Avoid type 7's and drink more water.
Type 2	Sausage-shaped but lumpy	You are a born leader, calm and unshakeable under fire. You have a knack for bringing others together for a plan. Avoid Type 7's.
Type 3	Like a sausage but with cracks on the surface	Your work ethic is impeccable and your hygiene beyond reproach. You are methodical in your plans, but work well on a team.
Type 4	Like a sausage or snake, smooth and soft	Well-rounded and diverse in your interests, life comes easily to you; remember to share your successes with others and avoid the traps of narcissism.
Type 5	Soft blobs with clear-cut edges	Active and 'on the go', you are flexible and improvise well. Your natural buoyancy keeps you afloat even in difficult times. Remember to slow down and take time for others.
Type 6	Fluffy pieces with ragged edges, a mushy stool	Artistic and imaginative, you are loyal to a fault. You are quick to make friends, but slow to leave a damaging relationship. Trust your instincts and go easier on the vegetables.
Type 7	Watery, no solid pieces. **Entirely Liquid**	You are a romantic and a dreamer; first to imagine and inspire, you are also quick to run when challenges appear. Your stool is abnormal and you should seek medical help.

The Daily Medical Examiner - medexaminer.wordpress.com

we have developed and moved on to urban lives, we now have no connection or contact with soil (dirt). According to him, we need to combine our modern lives with simple practices that kept us healthy and disease-free for many years. He recommends small, repeated exposures to dirt such as bacteria, plants, dust, soil and plant oils. This exposure also lets the good bugs to come into our system. Quite the opposite of what your doctor would suggest, correct? In turn, this strengthens our immune system and teaches our native gut colonies how best to interact with the world around us. We can do this by: (1) indulging with our pets (it has been said that those who have animals in their house have healthy inner ecosystems, i.e., good bugs); (2) spending more time outdoors (walk in the grass barefoot); (3) eating seasonal and local foods. Instead, we do the opposite: use sanitizers all the time, clean with chemicals and keep ourselves insulated in air-conditioned environments.

Allergies and asthma are a signal of the immune system breaking down; the precursor is usually an unhealthy amount of microorganisms in the first place, leading to an upset in the pH of the blood condition, which in turn affects immunity. Knight points out that several probiotics can relieve atopic disease and asthma, and certain microbe species can reverse food allergies or prevent them from developing in the first place. To sum it all up, he recommends: have a dog (start early, ideally prenatally) to help save your kids build up a healthy microbiome, avoid antibiotics early in life, perhaps take probiotics, and breastfeed. In general, exposure to different microbes, whether through older siblings, pets or livestock or through the good old-fashioned way of playing outdoors helps.

My patient Rahul always had an allergy. He said it was because of the external environment, and refused to believe it was his inner environment that was messed up. He had asthma, constipation, lethargy, insomnia and recently, weight gain. His body was screaming for a detox. When he met me, I could see his liver was completely off (based on the diagnoses of his organs), but he didn't seem to think so. He got diagnosed with jaundice three days after we met. He had not reached a complete full-blown stage of inflammation, but his constant allergy (which came in the form of sneezing, stuffed nose and sniffling all the time) was a sign that his body was breaking down from time to time. His jaundice diagnosis, in any case, meant he had to watch his diet carefully.

We first worked on his constipation by bringing in fermentation (about 20 per cent in the foods that he ate daily), providing a good probiotic supplement, including light, cooked foods with whole grain and vegetables, avoiding animal food and removing all the trigger foods (enumerated in Part Two of the book). He was also provided supplementation via herbs that would aid sleep and provide strength, e.g., *ashwagandha* and *shilajit* (talked about later). Sometimes a diet needs to be supplemented, since nutrients are not being absorbed due to poor bacterial support in the digestive system.

Jaundice did not leave him weak as he had been on the programme for three months; he was cleansed and ready to eat right to support the results he had seen in himself. His allergies came down to once in three months, which indicated he was on the mend. He had no constipation, was sleeping better and needed his Asthalin pump less frequently. He said he could feel himself 'flare up' as soon as he consumed dairy, sugar and junk.

Coeliac Disease

India is mainly a wheat-eating nation. In my practice, I have come to understand that sometimes, not always, we develop a resistance towards it. While gluten in whole wheat may work for me, it may not work for another person. Coeliac disease is an autoimmune disorder. A person suffering from it is intolerant to gluten, and it affects the small intestine. Zonulin, which is released by ingesting gluten, can be a big contributor to the tight junctions loosening in your intestines. If it leaks into your body via the intestines, it could, over time, play havoc with your immunity. It can develop at any age and at any time of your gluten-eating lifespan.

In a system with such an issue, the gut microbes have a hard time breaking down the gluten. It also increases malabsorption and therefore mal-digestion. Coeliac disease can predispose you to inflammation. It's a good idea to either check for gluten intolerance or watch out for bloating, flatulence, wheat belly (like a beer belly), heartburn, acid reflux and constipation after eating it.

This is what renowned poet, lyricist and screenwriter Javed Akhtar had to say after being on the diet for four months:

'As a matter of fact, for quite some time, I have been suffering from *Helicobacter pylori*. I had a bloated stomach and used to feel uncomfortable. A friend suggested that I meet Shonali Sabherwal. I came to know that my own daughter was under her care. She gave me a diet chart and told me to follow it for two months. It was not a difficult thing to do. I had to avoid dairy products, sugar, non-vegetarian food and gluten (white rice and wheat); brown rice was fine. I followed the plan and, lo and behold, it made a huge difference to my system. I was taking antibiotics and many other things, but I started feeling much more energetic. I would otherwise get tired in the afternoon. I started sleeping better. But my disease was not totally cured, so she suggested that I follow the diet again for two months since I had been such a good patient. I went away to the US and broke this regime, but I have started it again after coming back. I have lost weight, my waistline has reduced and I feel more energetic. More often than not we speak on the phone, she talks to my cook, and also sends products from her kitchen—it's a different kind of experience altogether. What is important is I lost weight, my stomach is in a better condition and I was not asked to starve—that's wonderful! To anyone who has the problem I have and wants to lose weight without starving, I suggest with total confidence that they contact Shonali.'

Fatty Liver—Is Your Microbiome Making You Toxic?

Most of us relate a fatty liver to alcohol, or maybe to an attack of jaundice. But a lot of people suffer from a syndrome called non-alcoholic fatty liver disease (NAFLD). In fact, most of my IBD, overweight, high-cholesterol, high-triglyceride and SIBO clients do. Anything above 5–10 per cent of your normal liver weight poses a problem. In such cases, since the liver stores sugar glucose, detoxifies blood (chemicals), stores nutrients, insulin and other hormones, all these functions get disrupted. When the liver gets overloaded, toxins recirculate in the system and start binding to protein, forming deformed molecules. When these deformed molecules make their way back to the liver, it has a hard time processing them. These toxins add to the inflammation, and since the liver handles hormones as well, there is an imbalance. Research on liver malfunction points us in the direction of bad gut microbes. In an article on 'The role of intestinal bacteria overgrowth in obesity-related nonalcoholic fatty liver disease,'[10] Ferolla et al. discovered that people who presented with obesity had an abundant overgrowth of the bad variety of bacteria and next to little or no presence of the good bacteria. According to the findings, the gut microbiota played a key role in the defence against pathogens by defending intestinal microvilli. Bacterial translocation (BT) due to a leaky gut interferes with blood supply to the liver. This blood contains products of digestion as well as microbial products derived from gut microbiota. This is one of the reasons for the disorder taking place in the liver. The paper also points out that cirrhosis and liver disease come about due to BT. Gut microbiota may also alter the bile–acid profile, contributing to liver disease. Both SIBO and obesity predispose one to NAFLD.

How Microbes Affect the Mind

'Your Colon Is a Great Reflection of Your Mind'

'Your brain . . .
weighs three pounds and has one hundred thousand miles of blood vessels.
contains more connections than there are stars in the Milky Way.
is the fattest organ in your body.
could be suffering this very minute without you having a clue.'

— David Perlmutter[11]

In my first book, I mentioned the connection between the gut and the brain. During foetal development, a part forms the central nervous system (CNS) and another the enteric nervous system connected via the vagus nerve. The enteric nervous system is located in the sheaths of tissue lining the oesophagus, stomach, small intestine and colon. Its nerve cells are bathed and influenced by the same neurotransmitters that influence your brain. The gut can upset the brain just as the brain can upset the gut.

Here is another connection: the vagus nerve. Vagus, which means 'wandering' in Latin, is the longest cranial nerve with multiple branches; the two main stems go down to the gut, passing through the neck and thorax, touching most organs along the way. It is also rooted in the brain (cerebellum). The 'gut instincts' we hear about often are those responses that start in the gut and travel to the brain. The vagus nerve acts like a walkie-talkie, streaming what's going on in the gut and organs, and sends it to the brain. The gut bacteria have a direct impact on the stimulation of cells along the vagus nerve. They actually act like hormones, sending messages to the brain via the vagus nerve.

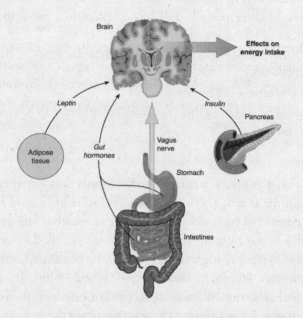

In a YouTube video,[12] Dacher Keltner of Berkeley University talks about the vagus nerve as being connected to a stronger immune response, oxytocin response (the cuddle hormone) and the inflammatory response of the body to disease—so it's a great mind–body nexus. A high level of activity in the vagus nerve was found to be directly linked to altruism, pro-sociality and more trust. The vagus nerve can be cultivated through mediation, breathing deeply into your abdomen (moving the diaphragm which send signals to the brain, which then sends neurotransmitters to every single cell in the body to relax), exercise and some stimulation on a daily basis. Here is one exercise to help you do it:

Take a deep breath, sucking in air for about four seconds, making sure the abdomen moves up (balloons out). Take another four seconds to slowly breathe out, letting the abdomen sink down this time (think of the navel drawing in towards the spine). Increase each breath in and out to five seconds. Reducing it to 5–6 breaths per minute creates cardio-resonance and will activate the vagus nerve. Cardio-resonance is the act of achieving a coherent heart rhythm. This happens because breathing patterns modulate the heart's rhythm. Breathing in this fashion also puts you in a calmer state of mind.

Good Gut Bite

In my first book, I highlighted how the brain relies on neurotransmitters such as serotonin, dopamine and norepinephrine to mediate moods. Of these, 80–90 per cent of serotonin, also called the 'feel-good' hormone, is made in the gastrointestinal tract, i.e., the gut.

In David Perlmutter's book *Brain Maker: The Power of Gut Microbes to Heal and Protect Your Brain*, he highlights that stress can be physical (from situations or an undue demand on the body) or on a dietary front (exposure to harmful toxins and pathogens). In both cases, we are exposed to a rush of extra blood to the heart (that's why your heart pounds faster), a release of excessive cortisol, adrenaline, and the release of inflammatory cytokines that send the body into an alert mode. Repeated stress can affect you over time and has been known to be one of the leading causes for nerve- and brain-related ailments like Parkinson's disease, multiple sclerosis, depression, dementia, Alzheimer's disease and autism.[13]

Our guts have their own immune system, referred to as gut-associated lymphoid tissue (GALT). Actually, this makes up 80 per cent, if not more, of the body's immune system. This is why our guts become so important. There is a transmission that happens between the immune system cells and your gut microbes constantly: this is the body's first response to anything that could go wrong in the gut. If you have good gut bacteria, they have the power to shut down excessive cortisol release—a precursor to systemic inflammation and immune system breakdown.

Perlmutter explains that Alzheimer patients' brains are in a state of inflammation, i.e., their brains are literally on fire. It is a fundamental element that underlies the development of Alzheimer's disease. Inflammation in the brain indicates cognitive decline and the start of dementia. Also, when comparing diseases of the bowel like Crohn's, ulcerative colitis, psoriasis, rheumatoid arthritis—all considered to be inflammatory conditions, some cytokines, i.e., proteins that affect the behaviour of cells, affect the inflammatory process. C-reactive protein interleukin 6 (IL-6) and tumor necrosis factor alpha (TNF-a) are all cytokines. TNF-a is a common factor that underlies all the conditions mentioned above and is found to be highly elevated in Alzheimer patients. Pharmaceutical companies are now developing ways to reduce this cytokine.[14]

Perlmutter, in his other book *Grain Brain*,[15] talks about the connection of elevated blood sugar levels to inflammation: elevated sugar levels in the blood promote toxicity if not used by the cells. A reaction called glycation is triggered, wherein sugar binds to proteins and certain fats, resulting in deformed molecules that don't function well. These molecules are called AGEs—advanced glycation end products—which set off inflammatory reactions. In the brain, sugar molecules combine with brain proteins to produce a lethal combination, contributing to the degeneration of the brain. The relationship between poor blood sugar control and Alzheimer's disease is so strong that researchers are calling it type-3 diabetes.

And gut microbiota is significantly affected by sugar. By itself, it causes a depletion in the good gut microbiota, and promotes bad gut microbiota; this in itself will cause the digestive systems to release an inflammatory response, initiating a decline in the health of the cells first in the digestive system, and then throughout the body. Diabetes patients, who have trouble with their insulin surges, will suffer a weakness wherever the nerves cannot transport the glucose, like in the legs (neuropathy) or the brain, ultimately damaging the nerves.

Now that we have established the connection between the various effects of gut microbes, let's move on to some crucial factors that are needed by the good microbes to survive.

The Importance of the Thymus Gland

Very deeply connected to the immune system, the thymus gland is a key factor when it comes to keeping our immunity up (see location in the picture). It produces a hormone called thymosin, which stimulates the production of disease fighting cells—also referred to as T-cells (certain kind of white blood cells). When the immune system starts turning against itself, which is what we call an autoimmune state, these cells help the body protect itself. It is protective of the endocrine and lymphatic systems (the defence network of the body).

THE ENDOCRINE SYSTEM

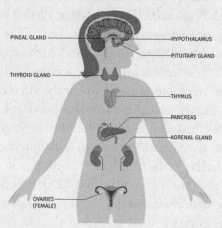

PINEAL GLAND

HYPOTHALAMUS

PITUITARY GLAND

THYROID GLAND

THYMUS

PANCREAS

ADRENAL GLAND

OVARIES
(FEMALE)

Good Gut Bite

Here Is an Exercise to Stimulate the Thymus

Make a fist with your right hand. Tap the area under your neck once, where the thymus gland is located (see picture), and follow it up with two quick taps in succession. Repeat ten times.

Can Your Poop Cure You?

As strange as it sounds, it can. Here is the strongest link between the microbiota you have and its relationship to your gut. A procedure called FMT (Fecal Microbiota Transplant) has been doing the rounds for a while now to cure various gut-related ailments. It is being used today as a remedial procedure to alleviate serious intestinal issues like ulcerative colitis and the like. So what happens? Basically, a stool sample is taken from a donor and introduced into the intestine of a recipient (i.e., the person suffering with the issue). It is introduced via a tube running from the nose to the gut, or the other way around from the rectum into the colon. The faecal material is first liquefied by adding saline in a blender and strained. It is then ready to be injected into the recipient. While it may sound awful, I felt it is necessary to bring out the latest developments in the medical world to treat serious ailments. This procedure points one in the direction of the power of gut microbiota to cure an ailment that otherwise does not respond to any other treatment.

Dr Avnish Seth, a gastroenterologist at Fortis Medical Research Institute (FMRI), has been conducting this procedure on a few patients who require it. In an article published by *DNA* (Maitri Porecha, 'One man's poop, another man's cure', *DNA,* 12 December 2016), Dr Avnish Seth says, 'It uses good bacteria from a healthy human gut to stabilize the colon fauna. While it has shown results, its long-term effects need to be observed.' A patient, Manas Shukla, has also set up a website, www.IhaveunoUC.com, after the transplant.

4

FOOD FOR THE MICROBIOTA TO FLOURISH

To prevent the good microbiota from dying and preserving the balance between the good and the bad, we must understand the crucial food elements at play before we move on to a discussion of how we would go about orchestrating a master detox diet. One of the largest influencers of our microbiome is diet.

The Reawakening to Fibre

Part of the imbalance in the inner ecosystems has happened because of the decline of fibre in our diets, specifically from plants. This includes whole grain, vegetables and legumes. The advent of modern food methods, influx of processed and refined foods, and the culture of eating out is now catching up with us. In India, we are shifting from a country that ate local and seasonal foods at home to one that is obsessed with Western lifestyle. Sadly enough, this has affected our gut diversity and caused the microbiota growth to decline. To add to this, the trigger foods (such as sugar, dairy, white processed flour [maida] and bad-quality fats [oils]) are a part of our day-to-day lives, feeding the bad gut microbes.

So while I have reiterated throughout how important fermentation is to introduce good transient microbes, it is prebiotic foods that feed these microbes. Fibre is another crucial component for maintaining good gut flora and fauna.

The Sonnenbergs term the right fibre as microbiota-accessible carbohydrates (MACs).[1] I travel all over, giving talks and hosting workshops. Everyone in the quest to stay slim has reduced the amount of carbohydrates in their diet. In my workshop for domestic cooks, when I ask cooks of different households what they prepare for their employers, more than 75 per cent of them say that they have excluded all carbohydrates (this includes MACs) from their homes. Then I jokingly ask them if everyone in the household is on a regular dosage of isabgol (Indian word for psyllium husk). The answer is 'yes', with a big grin on their faces. MACs are fibres the gut microbes can actually feed on to thrive and is a cornerstone of the macrobiotic approach. The stress is on whole grains (40–50 per cent of your daily volume consumption); vegetables (25–30 per cent of your daily volume consumption); legumes (10–15 per cent of your daily volume consumption); and fruits (5–10 per cent of your daily volume consumption). I eat a diet rich in complex carbohydrates from all the above sources, and include at least five fermented products a day. This forms the bulk of my main staples, the rest (nuts, seeds, decaffeinated beverages) go into the extras.

Demystifying Carbohydrates

Monosaccharides are the simplest carbohydrates, containing either glucose or fructose, i.e., a single molecule of sugar. They can be absorbed directly into the bloodstream from the digestive tract. Disaccharides (as the name suggests) are two monosaccharides linked together, namely, lactose and sucrose (sugar as we know it). Many monosaccharides linked together are called polysaccharides and are what we need, namely, complex carbohydrates. Most carbohydrates that are consumed in diets today, like white rice, pasta and bread, are simply starch and get absorbed before even hitting the large intestine. They convert into simple sugars (those that will throw your insulin levels off). MACs, on the other hand, get to your large intestine and feed your microbiota. Plant-based foods have over a thousand different MACs. Oligosaccharides consist of three to nine monosaccharides and are found in beans, whole grains, vegetables and fruits. These are fermented in the large intestine and release SCFAs.

Your gut microbes only respond to what you eat. You need to seriously think about what you are feeding it. How do you increase the MAC quotient of your meals? I mentioned earlier that the food that remains undigested moves after the first bulk of what you have eaten has been worked upon in the small intestine. The undigested foods move to the large intestine, which is actually where the microbes reside (larger colonies of them). A large portion of this undigested food is fibre. At this stage, the microbiota are looking out for MACs, and waiting for their food. Each species has a taste for different foods: some like bananas, while others like onions. Whatever we eat will help the microbiota multiply and, therefore, create balance for us.

Remember the theory of evolution and the process of natural selection put forth by Charles Darwin? This is how your microbiota survive. The ones that naturally reproduce multiply and are dominant. The gut is devoid of oxygen, and this proves to be the first challenge for the microbes. The Sonnenbergs further explain how they get energy in an oxygen-free environment. Cells need oxygen to reproduce. This is where the process of fermentation comes into play; the gut microbiota generate energy through this process. The second challenge is the speed at which digestion takes place. The rapid fermentation of MACs creates sort of an energy pool for these microbes. Here is where SCFAs are made. They provide energy to us when the fermentation takes place in our guts from the fibre we consume. As we absorb SCFAs into our tissue, our bodies remove the calories from the indigested fibre. In the end, we must boost SCFAs by eating foods rich in MACs. People consuming MACs and generating SCFAs actually lose weight, not to mention the reversal of leaky gut and inflammation.

The theory on Isabgol, aka psyllium husk

My dad took it every day; so does my brother. Both worked in the airlines, flying around the world. I guess with whacky flight timings and jet lag, poop habits get thrown off. However, don't confuse it with MACs. MACs are fibres found in plant-based foods, similar to whole grains, legumes, vegetables and fruits. Psyllium husk is just a supplement of fibre not accessible to microbiota and not fermented (ever wondered why after consuming it the faeces swells up and comes out?). It provides bulk and allows the stool to absorb more water, thus easing bowel movements. But it will not feed the microbiota and produce SCFAs.

So, for those low-carb dieters and constipated people out there, don't think a poop from psyllium husk is an indication that your stomach is doing well.

It is said that those with rich microbiome have more genes involved in generating health-promoting SCFAs.[2] Studies also point to the fact that meat-centred diets impact the microbiota. High-protein and low-carb diets decrease SCFAs; what they produce release more detrimental material in the colon.

PART TWO

5

WHY DETOX?

You may be wondering why you needed a whole explanation on the gut, the microbiota and the diseases that came from it to do a detox. As a health practitioner, I feel most people take detoxes very lightly. Tons of my clients call me to get a detox to get into a bikini or to lose weight. But a detox or cleanse is not about being so frivolous; it's a more serious approach to health and wellness. I could make it all very la-di-da and pretend these things could indeed happen overnight, but then I am setting you up for something worse on the immune system front later. That's why you should never go on a juice detox or a cooked detox that is not monitored by a health practitioner who is qualified to deal with you.

You detox because you need to balance your inner ecosystem and repair your gut. Even if you feel you are healthy and not suffering from any problem in your gut (my current situation), you can still go through a detox (every six months). The principle behind doing all the programmes highlighted in this book is to repair and rejuvenate; reverse leaky gut and inflammation; and to get on to a healthier eating plan. If you feel you fall in any of these categories, please go ahead and follow all the phases of this detox. However, if you feel you'd like to just do a mini-cleanse after having come back from a vacation or have somewhere to go and would like to feel and look better, you can do the juice or cooked detox diet.

From a macrobiotic perspective, eating sticky foods leads to sticky blood. Such foods include dairy, sugar, white flour, additives, processed foods and refined oils. By sticky, I mean blood that does not flow easily, but is sludgy and thick, even more acidic. Detoxes cleanse this blood and therefore become essential at least once a year. Let's not forget the importance of maintaining your health after this as well.

Detox—the very word means to cleanse oneself of toxins. I have played on this word to make it easier to remember its five different phases. These are:

reDEFINE

clEAN

rejuvenaTe

tOp it up

oXYGENATE

This is just a way to show how important each of these phases are for a thorough detox. Also, how long should a detox last? I specify the time frame of each phase to make a successful transition to the next. When you reach the third phase, rejuvenate, you have to stay there for four months to see a change (to see if your condition abates or reverses) or two months to make a difference (to make you feel good and clean from within).

Detoxes are highly personal and uplifting. If you are on a journey to clean up your gut and help the good microorganisms in your body, thereby impacting your blood condition and digestive health, it will also impact your inner energy, i.e., your *qi*, prana or life force. By this I mean that when toxins start to go out of your system, a lot of 'emotional' issues may come up as well. So make sure you are sensitive to yourself and those around you. Detoxes also take some time, so make sure you have the time for it in your life. Each phase will demand a certain way of eating, so either you or whoever cooks for you needs to be briefed. You must also keep aside time to pick up ingredients or get them organized.

6

REDEFINE

Phase 1—Duration: One Week

Redefine simply means to relook at your life at the moment vis-a-vis your food habits, food insensitivities and food choices, and look at why you crave foods.

In this phase, you will do three things:

(1) Keep a food diary: During this week, keep eating your current foods. But keep a food diary in the format shown below. Make a list of the foods you eat and what you drink from the time you wake up to the time you go to bed. This includes the sugar in your tea, the tea bags used, beverages consumed and all major and minor foods.

I would like you to also mention liquids, i.e., tea, coffee, sugar, soft drinks, etc. Do mention the ones in which you use sugar and milk. Make sure not to forget anything, even if you step out for a

	DAY 1	DAY 2	DAY 3	DAY 4	DAY 5	DAY 6	DAY 7
Breakfast							
Mid-morning							
Lunch							
Evening snack							
Dinner							
After-dinner snack							
After-workout snack							
Extras							

meal. I find that doing this just before I go to bed always helps.

(2) Check for food insensitivities: This is a good time to do the IgG blood test (mentioned earlier) that would rule out food intolerances (allergies). You can also be mindful of the following foods and watch yourself after you eat them: cow's dairy, gluten (in wheat), soy, eggs, anything with yeast or baking soda in it (bread, cakes, cookies, sauces, marmite). Pay attention to those foods or meals that made you feel bloated, gave you discomfort, gas, get you constipated (as a food may affect you for up to three days later), gives you itchy eyes, headaches, breakouts and/or an allergy.

(3) Why do you crave? I would also like to make you look at why and how you crave foods in this phase of redefining your future through the master detox diet. The macrobiotic approach has a wonderful way of explaining cravings and how they happen. If you look at the chart below, you see two polarities on each side termed as yin and yang. Basically, if any of you read my first book, *The Beauty Diet*, it outlines how the universal life force, prana or qi, is divided into two energies—yin and yang. This lends the character to foods as well. In foods, yang characteristics would be described as dense, contracted, drying, heating, salty; and yin characteristics as expansive, moistening, distending, sweet, cooling. This does not mean one is bad and one is good. But in foods, if we consume too much of the yin foods, we will try

to seek balance from the yang foods and vice versa. This is what leads to craving. What we need to do is to stop the craving cycle.

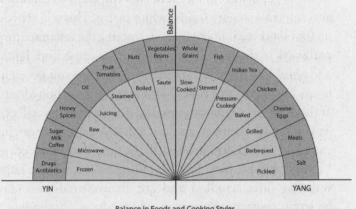

Balance in Foods and Cooking Styles

The best way that I could explain this is that if you have too much salt (yang), you always crave water (yin). If you look at the chart, too much sweet in your diet (sugar) will make you end up craving either another yang food like eggs, meats, cheese, salt or another yin food like coffee or dairy. The way to keep our cravings under check is to eat more foods mentioned on the chart in the centre. So if you have whole grains (natural complex carbohydrate sugars and fibre), which is a yang food, and include some vegetables that are yin, you will be in balance. If you are always eating from the two ends of the spectrum of yin and yang foods, you will set the cycle of craving in motion. So get ready to break the craving cycle.

Another appetite-related hormone is ghrelin (more yin), which stands opposite to leptin (more yang). When these two hormones do not behave well, your brain and stomach get disconnected. It makes you want to eat more, and you crave sugary foods (white carbs). This will set you up for blood sugar imbalances, triggering the inflammatory pathways in the body. Sleep deprivation cause both leptin and ghrelin to decrease, so please make sure you get eight hours of sleep at this time. Eliminate white carbohydrates at this time as continuous ups and downs in leptin will not let you know when you are satiated. If you are overweight, can't lose weight, feel stressed all the time, constantly crave 'comfort foods', have trouble falling asleep, have a large waistline (love handles) and are always tired, you may be leptin resistant. Your stomach produces ghrelin when it's empty; so if you want to lose weight, you want less of ghrelin (as it tells your brain you are hungry). Eating whole grains (brown rice and millets) at this time will help keep ghrelin under control.

Make a note in the extras section in your food diary after you look at the balance chart and determine which foods you include daily are fuelling your cravings. This phase is to redefine those crucial elements in your diet for the next phase.

Visualize Yourself: A Small Meditation

Consider this detox as a journey on healing yourself. Take out five to ten minutes every day to meditate and visualize what you are expecting from this detox.

(1) Sit quietly, cross-legged or on a chair (whatever works for you).

(2) Take deep belly breaths. Breathe in and expand your belly, and when you breathe out, push your belly back in. Some of you can bring your focus to the area under your nose, above the upper lip, just to narrow your attention (this is good for people who are anxious).

(3) Start going inward, from the top of your head down to your face, neck, shoulders, arms, torso (front), followed by your back, legs and feet. Now reverse the direction. Do this slowly, part by part, piece by piece.

(4) Ask yourself: do you feel stuck in any one area? If you do, don't linger there; just move on.

(5) Visualize yourself after the detox: how you are looking, feeling, glowing and smiling.

(6) Keep breathing deeply.

(7) Open your eyes and smile.

Activity: Write down what you are hoping to achieve through this detox journey on a piece of paper and stick it in a place where you can see it at least twice daily. Just remember, it connects you to the next phase. While you are doing this activity, you are putting a strong 'intention' out into the universe to see a positive change in your life and health. A detox is a great time to keep a journal and note down your feelings, as you will also start clearing up some negative emotions, personality traits and unwanted feelings.

Being addicted to sugar is as bad as, if not worse than, a smoking habit. This is a good time to question your 'relationship' with food. Why do you cling to certain foods like dairy? For example, dairy usually takes you back to your mother, as that's where you had the first taste of it. It is a 'comfort food' and you need to question your relationship with it and why you need such foods. Dairy makes for a sludgy blood condition (as explained earlier) and it will also make you stick to emotions and thoughts that do not define you, stagnating your energy. So this is the time when you will write down each food that you consume daily, and why you stick to them.

What to Expect out of Phase 1

The objective of Phase 1 is to kick-start and rev up your metabolism, make you question your relationship with unhealthy foods and lay the groundwork for the clean-out phase of your diet. If you follow the steps successfully, there is no reason why you will not meet with success. You may experience headaches, low moods, body odour, cold, cough, emotional outburst, allergies or any other discharges; and also experience withdrawals to foods that you will switch off from. This may happen if you have been a sugar eater, consume tea and coffee, and drink a lot of diet colas, etc. Just be in tune with your body, keep the visualization handy, and also note down the feelings you go through.

7

CLEAN

Phase 2—Duration: Ten Days (Three-Day Juice Detox and Seven-Day Cooked Detox)

In this phase, we have one objective: clean out the foods from your current diet that will cause the bad microbiota to multiply and add two detoxes, via a raw juice approach and a cooked approach.

Clean Out Dairy

If you really want to clean out, get rid of the dairy in your diet. Don't tell me you add only one teaspoon in your tea or coffee daily, I don't want to hear it. Just get rid of it. You can take a week to do it, but do it. To heal your gut (leaky gut), you need to remove these foods completely for a while. Not only does dairy trigger a rapid response to insulin but also creates an acidic blood pool and causes inflammation. Casein, a protein that is derived from dairy (cow's milk is 20 per cent whey and 80 per cent casein), does not assimilate into the digestive system. Think of casein going into your intestines and becoming like curd, sticking to its walls, thus preventing any chance of absorption. The processing of casein is slow and puts a further burden on a compromised digestive system. It has also been known to initiate cancer and cause deposits and cysts in the body. Milk's pH is 6.5, making it slightly acidic. When consumed, it is further warmed in our body, increasing the acidity levels. This creates a home for bad bacteria to thrive in, impacting the immune system. Homogenization alters the calcium levels and leads to loss of vital vitamins, while pasteurization increases the chances of milk putrefying and causing oxidation in the body, creating newer fat membranes with higher casein. Cow's milk has been declared as a pro-inflammatory food.

Clean Out Sugar

'Sugar is without question the number-one murderer in the history of humanity.'

—George Ohsawa

Recently, one of my contemporaries shouted out in every paper and magazine that sugar is actually good for you. She even called it the new superfood. I got a call from my friend (an eminent publisher of a leading group of magazines), saying, 'Has she lost the plot?' With all due respect, sugar—whether in your chai or in a dessert (be it Indian or Western)—is *bad* for you. How can one compare sugar to Ayurveda or yoga? And call something that will eventually kill you nectar? With

India being the diabetic capital of the world, can we really tout sugar as nectar and a superfood? As a health practitioner, I'm here to change lives, and I make sure that whatever I am saying is with 100 per cent confidence. So I am taking a stand on sugar (table sugar) in all forms being a killer.

Refined sugar, even if it comes from sugar cane, which we Indians use in our sweets, is a robber of everything: trace minerals, calcium and even thinking power. It causes a surge in insulin levels and irritability, leads to depletion of vitamin B12 stores, results in acidic blood condition, and most of all, leaky gut syndrome and inflammation as it feeds the bad gut microbiota and causes them to multiply.

Most of us would know this as a mantra by now, but I would like to revisit insulin 101 again: if blood sugar levels are thrown off with 'simple sugars', which include white rice, pasta, bread (all kinds, even multigrain has maida [processed white flour]), table sugar, sweeteners, (i.e., the easily digested starches), it will cause insulin levels to rise. This is because the body responds to sugar by releasing insulin, allowing the liver, muscles and fat to absorb sugar in the system that is swimming around. Until all of it has been utilized or stored away as glycogen, insulin will prevent the body from using fat as energy. If blood sugar levels stay high, cells reduce the insulin-responsive receptors on its surfaces; they become resistant to insulin. Insulin can keep knocking, but the cells don't hear them, and are unable to absorb glucose from the blood. The pancreas pumps more insulin to get cells to absorb the excess glucose in the blood. Then there is also type-2 diabetes (wherein the body cannot push glucose into cells) and other issues like heart disease, kidney failure, stroke,

Alzheimer's disease, etc. Sugar causes microbes to generate *Helicobacter pylori*, which drowns out the good microbes.

Good Gut Bite

On nutrition labels, watch out for:

- Treats that contain sucrose, maltose, glucose and fructose (anything ending in 'ose').
- Avoid anything with the word 'corn syrup': high-fructose corn syrup, corn syrup or organic corn syrup.
- Look out for sweeteners such as palm sugar, molasses, invert sugar syrup, cane and malt sugar.
- Watch out for products which scream 'sugar-free' and contain maltitol, xylitol, erythritol and sugar alcohols.

Many people ask me if jaggery is a substitute for sugar. Jaggery is sugar in its raw form, so it is a simple sugar that will convert slower but still impact the insulin levels. It is not to be consumed as an alternative to sugar on a daily basis. It should be a luxury food and diabetics should definitely not consume it. It will feed and multiply the bad gut microbiota.

Go back to the balance chart on page 83 of Part Two. Sugar and jaggery are yin—both are expansive in energy (they will cause energy to rise and hit your head, causing headaches). The upward-rising energy in the body always hits the head, leading to too much energy in the brain, which it cannot handle. This causes migraines, scattered energy, dissipated thinking, mood swings and anger. These will also cause your stomach to distend (expand). Inflammation is a product of expansion in the body: inflamed muscles can contract nerves, causing pain. Forget the scattered thinking, inflamed organs can even lead to chronic spasms and are a precursor to Alzheimer's disease, dementia, schizophrenia, not to mention premature ageing. We belong to the animal kingdom, so if we look at ourselves, we are yang contracted, i.e., dense in terms of bones, compact in terms of structure and heavier, compared to the plant kingdom, which is yin, i.e., expanded in terms of growth and lighter. We naturally seek foods to balance this contraction, so we seek sweet-tasting things that are yin in nature. Expansive tastes balance contraction, e.g., stress causes the body to contract. Many pilots, lawyers and investment bankers are heavy drinkers. Ever wondered why? Because alcohol is expansive and it releases all the contracted (yang) energy/ stress they have.

Here is how you can handle sugar cravings:

(1) Add a whole grain to your daily diet. By this I mean brown rice, sorghum (jowar), barley (*jav*),ragi (*nachni*), foxtail millet (*cheena*) and/or other millets. Chew these well.

(2) Eat one portion of protein at meals: fish, eggs (while on the rejuvenate phase of the diet) or chicken.

(3) Drink carrot juice daily. It brings in sweetness from the carrots (good-quality yin).

(4) Include sweet vegetables in your diet, such as red pumpkin (*lal kaddu/bhopla*), onions, cabbage and carrots.

(5) Add sprouts (steamed/boiled, not raw) to your diet; bring in the right plant protein to help regulate blood sugar levels like hemp protein or spirulina.

(6) Avoid artificial sweeteners and high-fructose corn syrup: they will make you crave more sugar.

(7) Include good fats like avocados, oily fish and nuts. These will keep you fuller longer.

(8) Adding chromium and balancing out your trace minerals helps (more on them later).

(9) Counteract cravings by increasing sour, pungent, spicy flavours in your foods.

(10) Cut back on salt, as eating too much of it will make you crave more sweet food.

(11) Cut back the consumption of eggs, cheese, meats and chicken if cravings are too intense.

(12) Cut back the consumption of dairy.

(13) Try and stay stress-free.

Clean Out Gluten

I do understand we are a wheat-eating nation, and while some of us maybe intolerant to gluten, others are not. But at this stage, getting it out of your current diet will certainly help. Gluten is found in wheat, barley (gluten analogue), rye and some grains; baked, processed products (processed meats, cold cuts); and sauces (look out for the labels that say gluten). It is used to hold together packaged products, so a reduced-fat product will have plenty of it (because no fat means there is nothing to hold it together). Gluten weakens the tight junctions of the intestine. So, if you stay off it, the body may have a chance to start closing the loose junctions in the intestinal wall. If, however, it is in your diet and leaks into your system, you will develop antibodies to it, and will eventually lead to inflammation.

Good Gut Bite

Watch out for hidden gluten in the following packaged products:

- Tomato sauce
- Soy sauce
- Salad dressings
- Cooking sprays
- Ground spices
- Mayonnaise
- Anything with added flavours
- Stock cubes (vegetable or chicken)
- Frozen foods
- Creamer
- Ready-made gravy mixes

Note: Read all the ingredients on products you buy.

Clean Out Grains (Just for Two Weeks of This Phase)

For two weeks, include no grain in your diet. In the third week, you can add brown rice and millets (*kodo*, barnyard, cheena, i.e., foxtail millet). This is because the bad microbes will feed on anything with sugar and starch in them, and for two weeks, I would like to starve the bad bacteria before introducing the good microbiota-accessible carbohydrates (MACs) in the diet, for a master detox plan later. I am going with the assumption that most of you want a good detox and would like to get rid of the bad microbes you are harvesting.

Popularly known as FODMAPs, some foods are fermentable oligo-, di-, monosaccharides, and polyols. Saccharide is another name for sugar. Oligosaccharides, disaccharides and monosaccharides are all sugars. Polyols are sugar alcohols. Some people lack the enzyme to break down lactase (a disaccharide), which means they cannot digest dairy and are lactose intolerant. Yet others cannot break down fructose (an oligosaccharide), producing problems in the gut. When such foods pass into the large intestine undigested, they create issues. If your digestive system is compromised, especially if you suffer from small intestinal bacterial overgrowth (gas, bloating and pain, especially after eating grain or sugary meals is a sign), it is best to avoid these FODMAPs at this stage. For those who are doing this programme as a general cleanse and have a strong digestive system, including the whole grains mentioned above is fine. You may limit them and not remove them entirely. Limiting short-chain carbs at this stage will help you detox better, if you do react to sugars. However, with FODMAPs it's relative as to what one can handle. Only you will be able to say if you react to them. FODMAPs include garlic, onions, black beans, baked beans, chickpeas, kidney beans, mushrooms, mung beans, soybeans, amaranth flour, barley flour, bran cereals, wheat, wheat germ, semolina, avocados, apples, apricots, custard apple, dates, figs, guava, lychee, mango, peaches, pears, pineapple, pomegranate, prunes and watermelon.

I know at this point you might be wondering, 'What do I eat then?' The answer is: vegetables, fruits and legumes (limit if following the FODMAPs list). Include low-starch vegetables like cabbage, green peppers, broccoli, snake gourd (*chichinda*), okra (*bhindi*), bottle gourd (*doodhi*), celery, leafy greens, onions, leeks, mushrooms, radish, cucumber, eggplant, snow peas, bok choy, tomato, zucchini, cauliflower and most Indian vegetables that are in season. Stick to minimal use of starchy vegetables like sweet potato, red pumpkin, peas and corn. I like to keep a vegetarian approach at this point due to the less time required for digesting vegetables, the objective being to free up digestive energy. I reiterate that this is only for this phase.

Note: Okra (bhindi) and eggplant should be minimized.

Clean Out Unhealthy Fats

By unhealthy fats, I mean hydrogenated and trans-fats. These usually come via processed and refined foods such as biscuits and Indian fried savoury products like *khakra*, soy *chakli*s, nachni chips and *chivda*. They are used in these products as they extend shelf life. They definitely promote inflammation. Cell walls are made of fat, and therefore they need healthy fats to absorb nutrients from your bloodstream and prevent toxins from entering them. Cut down on your intake of saturated fats from dairy and meats (this again is just for this phase of the diet) and refined cooking oils, which will skew the omega-6 to omega-3 ratio and lead to inflammation (explained later in detail). Unhealthy fats feed the bad microbes, the ones that will cause harmful pathogens to propagate themselves and cause mutation of cells, leading to inflammation. For example, most refined oils say they are fortified with omega-6. However, too much of this type of fat is pro-inflammatory, so avoid concentrated sources of omega-6 oils. Anything that says 'partially hydrogenated fats', 'trans-fats', 'interesterified fats', 'high-stearate' or 'stearic-rich fat' should be avoided. Also, avoid all refined oils made from corn, peanut, palm, safflower, soybean and sunflower. While I do understand that most of us are using refined oils for our Indian way of cooking, I would urge you to go in for blends that are less refined, which means you have to pay a little more. But since we use it daily, we need to look for superior-quality brands.

Good Gut Bite

The Good Fats

Any good cold-pressed oil, like sesame, coconut, mustard, flaxseed, palm, olive, and nuts, seeds, avocado and ghee. Why do I not mention butter here?

After much research, I have come to the conclusion that butter actually works if it is from grass-fed cows as it contains more omega-6. In that case, it works like ghee, even though it comes from a dairy source. Butter is pure animal fat with traces of dairy protein (the stuff I have been saying is harmful for you). It would be wise to keep it out of this phase. Think of including it later in the rejuvenate phase of the plan.

Mark Hyman in his book *Eat Fat, Get Thin* advocates the use of grass-fed butter. He says the cow's stomach ferments vitamin K1 (found in leafy greens) into vitamin K2, which then shows up in the dairy fat. Vitamin K2 is important for bone and heart health. Grass-fed butter also contains a fatty acid butyrate (found in ghee as well) that promotes intestinal health and fights inflammation throughout the body.[1]

Clean Out Alcohol

Alcohol produces 'empty sugars' and has pretty much the same effect as sugar in the body, i.e., it impacts insulin levels much the same way. Alcohol (if you look at the balance chart) comes under yin foods and is very expansive. It will cause you to crave more sugar. Your body will try to balance the effect and cause you to reach for more eggs, meat or baked products. It also inhibits certain enzymes that help fight inflammation. The sugars from alcohol will also feed the bad microbiota in your gut, causing them to multiply. Since we are in a clean-out phase and are trying to mitigate the effects of bad bacteria in the gut, we must remove anything that will multiply it at this point. When I had candida, even a glass of wine would cause my symptoms to get worse, and I would suffer for a long period after that.

Clean Out Antibiotics and Painkillers

Antibiotic literally means 'against life'. Discovered about seven decades ago, it has become the cure for all ailments. These are prescribed even for a simple cold or fever, not allowing the body to fight off the problem with its own healing powers. Antibiotics not only kill colonies of microbiota, but like chemotherapy, they don't distinguish between good and bad microbes/cells and kill them all en masse. This allows the unfriendly bad microbes to take over completely. So if you are the kind that pops pills at the drop of a hat, you need to come up with alternative ways of dealing with your illness—through home remedies or homeopathy—and reduce the use of antibiotics. You also need to reduce pain medication (aspirin or ibuprofen), if you are taking any, as it destroys the mucosal lining of the intestines, leading to more inflammation and weight gain.

Good Gut Bite

Natural Painkillers

- Arnica: This is a homeopathic remedy known to fight pain, injury, sprains, etc.

- Ginger compress: Grate ginger the size of a lime, squeeze juice in a pan of boiling water, wrap the piece of ginger in a muslin cloth or hanky and drop into the pan like a tea bag. Take two small hand towels, dip it in water and apply on pain areas like you would do a compress. Keep repeating this using the other towel.
- Craniosacral therapy: This is a biodynamic therapy, tapping into the cerebrospinal fluid which bathes and nourishes the brain and nervous system, and helps in healing your condition (source provided at the end of the book).

Clean Out Eggs

The energy of eggs as per the balance chart is extremely yang and doesn't augur well for a digestive system that is at present in recovery mode. So I would clean out the eggs. Eggs become a reactive food in this phase, and we do not want the body to trigger off an inflammatory response. They are not easy on the digestive systems of those people who suffer an imbalance in their inner ecosystem. I see most women on high-protein diets (on a weight-loss/fit plan) having 6–8 egg whites a day; most of them have severe constipation or some gut issue going on. Eggs are not good in this phase of your plan.

Clean Out Diet Sodas and Sweeteners

People who take diet drinks generally tend to compensate by overeating. Diet sodas increase appetite and make you hungrier. The combination of aspartame and carbonation signals reward centres in the brain, including dopamine. This increased activation triggers hunger responses. To top it all, artificial sweeteners disrupt the microbiota in the gut. Aspartame also breaks down as formaldehyde, which is likely to cause cancer. Sucralose will cause insulin reactions as well. In a study conducted by Jotham suez et al. in March 2014 on artificial sweeteners,[2] it was concluded that non-caloric artificial sweeteners induced dysbiosis and glucose intolerance. In another study, it was found that sweeteners could not be fermented by the gut microbiota and led to a disruption in microbial diversity.

Clean Out Anything That Multiplies—'Bad Bugs'

In addition to diet sodas, stay away from beverages; refined and processed foods; refined carbohydrates in the form of white rice, pasta, bread, cookies, biscuits and cakes; sauces; anything with preservatives; fruit juices; coffee; honey; and Indian tea and coffee. Exposing yourself to environmental toxins, e.g., by using household cleaners, eating foods which are not organic and not washed properly, and having genetically modified foods will add to the bad-bug load.

Checking with your doctor to remove parasites, if you may have any, is a good idea in this phase. Also make sure that you wash the vegetables and greens that are not organic in one tablespoon of vinegar and half a teaspoon of salt (per kilogram).

Clean Out Yeast

Just remember that yeast feeds yeast. If you have a digestive condition, you already have yeast (colonies of bacteria, not good ones) in your gut and body as well. You cannot have anything made with yeast to multiply it. Bread, cakes, cookies, alcohol, marmite and some vinegars fall in this category.

Clean Out Table Salt

Add rock or sea salt, and throw away the regular table salt (refined). It is high in chemicals and 99.5 per cent of it is sodium chloride, dextrose (sugar), potassium, iodine and the like. It has been stripped off all mineral content, and apart from giving you water retention and high blood pressure, it does nothing on a nutritional front. Rock and sea salt are alkaline, and they help neutralize the effects of acid-forming foods. They retain all their mineral content. Good-quality salt, in turn, will actually strengthen digestion and help with bowel movements. The right salt will help the process of detoxification easily via kidneys. Those who suffer from hypothyroidism can use iodized sea or rock salt.

Clean Out Stress

When you are under stress, the body releases cortisol in excessive amounts. It should help you out, but it ends up harming you if the body cannot deal with it. For one, it switches on inflammation when produced in excess and does the opposite when just the right amount is produced. High levels will make you age faster and low levels will cause adrenal fatigue. Since we are talking about 'cleaning out the stress', let's also talk about the thyroid and how it affects this master gland.

The Cortisol and Thyroid Connection: Why Are So Many People Suffering from It Today?

I'd like to talk about this subject here, not only because it is imperative on a 'gut level' but also because it is deeply connected to the thyroid epidemic our nation is facing. High cortisol levels change the strains of the bacteria in the gut and also increase gut-lining permeability. This happens as cells in the gut as well as the immune system trigger certain chemicals (when you are under stress), which are pro-inflammation. Stress and food for like the chicken-and-egg story, one is always trying to figure out which came first. Here is my opinion: We have made the connection between your gut microbiota and the brain in Part One. The gut is your second brain and responds to everything you are eating and thinking. It is the inner engine where food combustion happens, symbiosis takes place between the foods and gut microbiota (good and bad), and nutrients are extracted. To me, it is obvious that it would influence your brain.

One of my clients who has ulcerative colitis would constantly complain that she was not losing any weight. She felt the diet was not working and kept telling me how fed up she was. I tried to explain to her that inflammation in the gut, coupled with an autoimmune ailment, was not going to make her shed weight. We needed to tackle her gut first, then the weight. But she was impatient and at the same time not even 60 per cent diet-compliant.

At the end of four months, I was pretty stressed myself, so much so that I got anxious every time I was to meet her. I knew the yelling, screaming and tantrums were a result of her gut condition, and she couldn't help being this way. Without taking names, I tried to talk to my close friend about it, and he thought I should walk away for being treated this way all the time. My psychologist advised me the same. But since I take the job of a 'healer' very seriously, I continued to act with compassion all the time (thank God for vipassana meditation). She would yell, and I would listen, praying that someday her condition would turn around. I knew the stress in her gut caused her mood swings; this was the inflammation in her brain talking as well.

If you have a thyroid condition, this section will clear your doubts about the chicken-and-egg story. As you say, did your hormones go out of order, or did you get it because you were stressed? Did the gut microbiota get disrupted before, and were you already in a state of dysbiosis? Let's connect the dots.

The adrenal glands, also known as the 'glands of stress' (see location in page 67), help the body cope with the onslaught of stress. The adrenals act as control organs for your flight-and-fight response. Many hormones are produced here: oestrogen, pregnenolone, adrenaline, progesterone, testosterone, dehydroepiandrosterone (DHEA), aldosterone and, most important of all, cortisol. The adrenal and thyroid connection originates in the brain. The thyroid's main job is to produce the right amount of thyroid hormone to tell your cells how fast they should burn and produce proteins. The adrenal glands' main job is to produce the right amount of stress hormones to help you respond to all kinds and degrees of stressors. Think of the adrenals and thyroid as guardians or protective intermediaries of the endocrine (hormone-producing) system. They relay information back and forth between the brain and the body. The signalling for the release of both hormones originates in the brain (hypothalamus), which sends messages to the pituitary. From here, hormonal messages are relayed to both the thyroid and the adrenal glands. They, in turn, produce hormones and provide feedback to the brain that says 'this is good for now'. A big adrenal response to a highly stressful event is normal, but then the adrenals also need to rest. However, I see that people these days don't reach a point where they aren't stressed. Thus, we keep forcing our adrenals to constantly respond, without any rest. You need just the right amount of cortisol for the thyroid to function optimally. Too much (from acute stress) or too little (as a result of continuous stress over time) can lead to problems. With constant stress, the thyroid hormone production is reduced, and the loops (which are responsible for transmitting messages between the thyroid and adrenals) get disrupted. This leads to an imbalance in the hormones produced by both parts, which results in the following symptoms:

(1) Fatigue
(2) Sluggishness
(3) Weight gain
(4) Poor concentration
(5) Hair loss
(6) Memory loss
(7) Intolerance to cold
(8) Infertility

High cortisol levels will show up as:

(1) Not waking up fresh, but sluggish in the mornings (called 'rising cortisol')
(2) Fatigue
(3) Facial lines
(4) Low sexual drive
(5) Sugar cravings
(6) Caffeine cravings
(7) Weight gain in the middle (most men have this around the belly)
(8) Low immunity levels

The interplay between thyroid and adrenals takes place over time; it doesn't happen all of a sudden. When I had a lot of work stress at one point in my life and was not taking care of myself, my teacher Warren Kramer told me, 'Shonali, you will blow your thyroid gland, as it is the only thing which blows under pressure.' Some people may not have it reflected in their tests, but they will remain in a subclinical hypothyroid state, experiencing symptoms of low thyroid.

Good Gut Bite

Tips for Breaking the Cycle

Get a high-quality multivitamin + mineral complex containing selenium, iodine, iodized salt, and vitamins A, B, C and E, which are all necessary in the production of thyroid hormones, i.e., for an underactive thyroid. I believe in getting it via foods, so you can also include kombu or Japanese seaweed (available in India, see Source List) in your dahls or beans—a piece the size of your nail is enough for one person. Add when the dahl/bean starts cooking, i.e., when you put the water in it, and remove it when *tarka* (tempering) is done.

(1) Eat to support your thyroid: Use the rejuvenate (next) phase to set your diet right. Focus on breakfast, eat at regular mealtimes, include quality protein in each meal and snack, and clean out caffeine.

(2) Sleep: Set a reasonable time for bed and stick to it; 10 p.m. is ideal. Allow yourself enough time to unwind. I used to be extremely sleep-deprived, and worked really hard on this aspect of my life. I dimmed the lights in the house, lit an oil infusion with lavender in my room, moved the television out of my room, kept the phone away and did not answer calls after 9 p.m. (unless urgent), and did

not take the laptop to bed. This helped me put the adrenals in a forced state of rest.

(3) Manage your stress: Resort to cortisol elevators like yoga, meditation, tai-chi, deep breathing, massage and exercise.

What to Expect Out of Phase 2

Phase 2 is a great time to actually clean up your diet and start laying the foundation for everything good that is to come. This phase will begin to balance your inner ecosystem, getting rid of unwanted microbes and not multiplying the bad ones. You will have steadier blood sugar levels. Therefore, you can expect to feel lighter, clearer in your head and calmer. You will no longer have any cravings and will have better bowel movements. You may also be able to kick off persistent allergies or recurring headaches, or some condition that has afflicted you for very long.

Additionally, Watch Out for These Contaminants

(1) Mercury in fish: Mercury is a chemical that worked its way up the food chain, straight into the sea. Plants in the sea contaminated with mercury are consumed by small fish, which are then consumed by larger fish. These end up in you if you are a fish eater. I once met a guy at Kushi Institute who was

there because he had mercury poisoning; it had damaged his nerves and brain. So all we can do is minimize it in our diets, though eating fish has its own array of health benefits. I would also advise replacing any mercury fillings that you may have in your teeth. Old-school dentistry used only mercury for fillings. I've had mine replaced.

(2) Plastic: It contains a chemical called bisephenol-A (BPA). Water bottles, plastic storage containers and plastic bags (so glad our government got rid of those) contain these. BPA leeches into your food and water to contaminate you over a period of time. It has been known to mimic oestrogen, by binding on to oestrogen-receptor sites, causing disruption in the hormone. Many studies have linked it to polycystic ovary syndrome (PCOS), abnormal births and thyroid issues. Cut out the plastic for sure.

(3) Genetically modified organisms (GMOs): Say no to GMOs for sure. Not only are they created artificially but also grown in soils stripped of nutrition and full of pesticides. It definitely kills of our good microbes. Moreover, pesticides have been linked to coeliac disease and autoimmune conditions.

(4) Household cleaners: All of them are doused with chemicals and volatile organic compounds (VOCs). I stick to citronella oil to clean my floors.

Medication	Supplement With
Antibiotics	A good probiotic: Enterogermina, Econorm, VSL #3, B vitamins, vitamin K, magnesium, calcium, coenzyme Q10
Diabetic	Vitamin B12, coenzyme Q10
Pain Medication	Iron, folic acid, vitamin C, calcium, magnesium, selenium, vitamin D
Blood pressure	Vitamins C, B1, B6, calcium, magnesium, sodium and zinc
Cholesterol	Coenzyme Q10
Thyroid	Calcium

Food Item	Substitue With
Breakfast cereal	Home-made *poha*, home-made granola
Commercial bread	Unyeasted or sourdough bread or roti /chapatti
Chips	Home-made chips (oven)
Coffee	Herbal tea, decaffeinated coffee
Cookies	Home-made with almond flour or gluten-free flour, no yeast
Dairy	Almond milk, peanut milk, rice milk, coconut milk
Dips	Guacamole, hummus, salsa, chutney
Drinks	Carrot juice, *kanji*, rejuvelac, kombucha, kefir, green tea with stevia
Burgers	Home-made burger with fish/chicken/ vegetarian with whole wheat bun
Ice cream	Dairy-free home-made ice cream
Milk chocolate	Dark chocolate (75 per cent and above)

Pasta/noodles/ spaghetti	Buckwheat, quinoa, vegetable or gluten-free
Pizza dough	Home-made thick pizza base with gluten-free flour (made firm on *tava* or oven)
Sugar	Stevia, fruit pulp, fruits, dates
Whey protein powder	Vegan protein, pea protein powder or brown rice protein powder

8

REJUVENATE

Phase 3—Duration: Four Weeks after the Clean Phase (May Take Up to Twelve Weeks, Depending on the Severity of the Gut Healing Required)

This is the most important phase of your plan. It involves changing some deep-rooted underlying issues in the gut and replenishing it with a solid inner ecosystem—building the bedrock of repair for the gut lining and good microbes, and reversing any issue you'd like to resolve. This is where the master detox diet will come into reality. Besides following the principles of clean-out from Phase 2, you will add the following foods outlined in this phase. This is the whole shebang. To make this plan successful, we must start adding the following foods. I have listed them below:

1. Add Microbiota Accessible Carbohydrates (MACs)

In this phase, in addition to whole grain, the diet will centre around vegetables, legumes and fruit, and in smaller quantities, chicken, meat and fish (if you are non-vegetarian). MACs, as discussed earlier, are carbohydrates found in plant-based sources of foods. The more MACs you consume, the more fermentation will take place in your gut, and the more SCFAs you will produce. While there is a theory on which MACs to introduce, I prefer to adopt generics in this phase. It is very hard to find out which strains of gut microbes dominate your gut individually, so it's best to follow the path of least resistance and adopt a middle path when introducing MACs. It is also not possible to measure the MAC content in foods, like you would do for protein, carbohydrates and fat.

MAC 1: Whole Grain

We Indians have not yet understood the power of this food group. As a health practitioner and an opinion leader in this field, I take my spoken and written word very seriously. So be rest assured that I don't recommend whole grains lightly.

As the Sonnenbergs explain,[1] anything that is milled has less fibre or MAC content than something that is 'whole'. The same was espoused by my teachers at Kushi Institute. For example, removing the bran and germ from wheat (wheat is made of endosperm, i.e., germ + bran), as opposed to keeping it whole, reduces its MAC fibre. In my opinion, brown rice is the only whole grain that has a high MAC content, similar to a whole millet (like foxtail millet).

My recommendation in this phase would be to stick to an intact whole grain. In the Indian markets, that leaves us with brown rice and whole millets (i.e., barley [jav], sorghum [jowar], finger millet [nachni or ragi] in its 'whole' form, not milled into a flour). Avoid wheat and barley at the moment due to their gluten content. We can reintroduce these later, in the next phase. It always helps to dry roast millets first before boiling. For one, they cook better, and two, roasting removes the allergens and other irritants, if any. So try to minimize grain flours and eat the grain in its whole form. I say this for people who may find it difficult to have a whole grain for two meals. If you'd like to eat chapattis, then go ahead and add bran to the flour (oat bran or wheat bran).

MAC 2: Vegetables

Focus on all vegetables, especially on dark leafy greens, squash, sweet potato, peas (not if you don't digest them well), Brussels sprout (Indians don't use this vegetable a lot, but it's available), lotus stem (*kamal ki kakdi* or *bhen*) and avocados. In dark leafy greens, go beyond spinach, amaranth (*cholai*) and fenugreek (methi). One leafy green to explore which has more fibre than any of these is Malabar spinach, also called *pui shaak* (Bengali), *mayalu* (Marathi) or *valchi bhaji* (Konkani). These vegetables make my microbiota happy. Also important are brassica vegetables, which have been studied for their high concentrations of glucosinolates, a natural compound in pungent plants known to be anti-carcinogenic. These include broccoli, cauliflower, cabbage, kale, summer squash (yellow, looks like zucchini), regular squash (*lal kaddu* or *bhopla*), turnips (*shalgam*) and kohlrabi (*ganth gobi* or *nool kol*, better known as *kadam* in Kashmir [known for kadam saag]).

MAC 3: Fruits

All fruits are great, but stressing on bananas is good as they are prebiotic and the microbiota loves them. For those who tend to have acidity and an excess build-up of mucous (coming out of any orifice of the body), don't include bananas, apples, berries (blue/black), pears and oranges. You will see in the diet section that I have used a lot of combinations in juices and smoothies.

MAC 4: Legumes

Legumes/beans have got a bad rap for causing indigestion, and you are probably saying the same thing if you do have a gut issue going on. By these I mean kidney beans (red/black), white beans (*lobhia/raungi*), green mung and black beans (*kaala masur*). However, they are loaded with good fibre that your microbiota loves.

To make them more digestible, as I mentioned earlier, add kombu (see the Source List), a seaweed that is available in India. All you have to do is add a nail-sized piece of it when your beans start to cook and then remove it when it is done. They predigest the bean. Kombu in itself is a high source of dietary fibre and has been known to be a prebiotic and an MAC as well.[2]

MAC 5: Nuts and Seeds

I would include all of them, specifically walnuts, almonds, pistachios, Brazil nuts, cashews, and sunflower, pumpkin and flaxseeds, and minimize peanuts.

> ## Good Gut Bite
>
> ### Ways to Sneak Fibre into Your Diet
>
> - Add bran to your smoothies.
> - Think fibre when you think of snacks.
> - Increase your intake of fruits and vegetables.
> - Change whites to browns, e.g., white rice to brown.
> - Have a bean salad daily.
> - Have a shaker handy with a mix of flaxseeds, sunflower and pumpkin seeds.
> - Sprinkle seeds over dairy-free yogurt (or yogurt in the top-it-up phase of your detox).

2. Add Healthy Fats

Healthy fats can be derived from monounsaturated sources like avocado, sesame, flaxseed, olive and canola. If they are cold-pressed, it is even better. Also add the omega-3 fats from oily fish and walnuts. Flaxseeds and walnut oils are high in omega-3, which will use fatty acids to build anti-inflammatory compounds as well as create a whole new set of molecules that fight inflammation.

Oily Fish

If you eat fish, it's a good time to add it here in this phase. Protein makes you feel fuller and satiated, and increases thermogenesis (the amount of calories you burn when ingesting your food). Eating good-quality protein will increase your metabolic rate as well. Fish increases blood levels of tryptophan, a precursor to serotonin (the happy neurotransmitter). Good fish are mackerel (*bangda*), Indian salmon fish (*rawas*), sardines (*pedvey*) and herring (*hilsa*).

If you are vegetarian, add a fish-oil supplement (with 650 mg of EPA and DHA combined) or include chia and flaxseeds in your diet (two tablespoons a day).

While these food groups form the bulk of your meals, we cannot neglect the power of bringing in fermentation, to up the good microbiota. This is my favourite part of the book.

3. Add Probiotics

A Microbial Act of Balance

I remember my Ayurvedic doctor, Dr Soumit, saying, 'If you don't have some mucous, how will the wick burn strong?' We need some amount of mucous, but when gut dysbiosis occurs, there is too much in the system. This acts as a barrier that does not allow microbes to go too close to the mucosal lining. It also serves as food for the gut microbes, as it has remnants of the carbohydrates we have eaten. If we are starved of microbial diversity, this mucosa does not function at its optimal condition. Therefore, to prevent disease, we must be able to balance our gut with the right microbes. However, we all have different microbes, and one size does not fit all.

This is why kefir, a probiotic drink with good microbes, may benefit a person with allergies, but may not work on someone else with IBD. Even a generic probiotic drug may not work for two people in the same manner. I see a lot of people consuming drinks and products just because someone is touting them as healthy, but it is important to consider your own condition (which only a health practitioner can assess) before consuming these drinks or products.

The endeavour is to push the microbiota to constantly produce SCFAs that also produce T-regulatory cells and other important hormones that balance the immune system's response. I have yet to come across a diet other than the macrobiotic diet that stresses on gut microbes and enhances the diversity within to impact overall health and the outward manifestations of it. There is significant evidence as documented in all the references cited in this book itself of benefitting from working out a cocktail of good microbes for you and increasing diversity in your gut. I can assure you that most doctors and dieticians (seeking to make you lose weight or work with health concerns) will only prescribe you a probiotic and not know how to orchestrate the increase in good gut microbes through your food. You will have to turn to someone who practises a more holistic approach and understands constitution.

While some bacterial populations are residents in our guts, probiotic bacteria do not live in our gut, they come and go. It's important that your body has these at all times. So, incorporate them into your gut along with a good diet plan. The probiotic bacteria communicate with the resident bacteria when they visit, impacting immunity positively.

I don't remember the last time I fell sick with a cold, cough or fever. It's because I consume up to five fermented products daily. I also remember that during the launch of my first book, *The Beauty Diet*, when many people saw Jacqueline Fernandez, Neha Dhupia and me on stage, they said our skin was glowing. I attribute it to the way we were all eating and the plethora of fermented foods in our diets. The benefits of good fermentation are tremendous, and its impact fortifies your immunity to a hitherto unknown level.

Good Gut Bite

How Gut Bacteria Influence Your Food Choices

I often tell my friends that the more 'clean' I am, the less I want to go towards unhealthy choices. In essence, what does that mean? The healthier my gut and blood condition are, the higher the 'vibrational' energy that I am creating to attract the right foods (also circumstances, people, situations) in my life. Underlying the right food choices are my gut microbes (bacteria) that guide this process, and want foods that will make them thrive and grow. Remember the vagus nerve? The gut bacteria manipulate neural signals along this nerve and influence what we crave and feel. They have the ability to change our feelings, how we taste our food, absorb nutrients and release toxins. This is all done not selflessly but selfishly to propagate their own species.

Add Fermentation: Your Weapon Against Bad Bugs and Mucosal Lining Boosters

Come one and all, this is a story to tell,
To give you a peek into every healthy cell,
How fermenting your foods is panacea for health,
That which will lead you to abundant wealth,
It's the tiny good bugs that hold it together,
Your lifelong friends—not only in fair weather.

History of Fermentation in India

As Indians know it today, fermentation via our diets is added through yogurt (dahi), buttermilk (*chhach*) and pickles (made using lots of spices and refined vegetable oil) every day. A sweet substance known as soma and *sura* (wine/beer) were the first fermented products made in India by Vedic Aryans (c. 1500 BC). Soma was a plant-based product made using the juices of plants and barley. In the Rig Veda, it is mentioned that this mix was fermented for fifteen days. Sura, on the other hand, appears in the Yajur Veda. It was prepared with germinated paddy, germinated barley and parched rice. Yeast was used as a fermenting agent. The use of dahi or yogurt (origins 6000 to 4000 BC) is also mentioned in the Rig Veda. Different methods were used to make it, with one book mentioning a recipe using whey and rice milk. In south India, fermented food is included in the daily diet through idlis, dosas or appams. Similarly, in north India, around the time of Holi, the fermented drink kanji is very popular. Darker carrots are used to make it, because before the seventeenth century, only the darker ones were available until farmers started using hybrids. This variety is also used for the anthocyanins present in them, which have health-boosting, anti-inflammatory and antioxidant properties.

In the post-Vedic period, different agents were added for fermentation. In whole grains, rice and barley were used; in fruits, grape, palm, mango, wood-apple; and in agents, sugar cane, lime, liquor and honey. I have dealt with this topic to paint a picture on fermentation in our Indian culture which dates back to our ancestors.

Microorganisms Everywhere

Fermentation takes place all around us. Microbial cultures are important to our life's processes—not only what they do within us but also how they come into play around us. We have in reality descended from these microorganisms. They are our lineage, our connection to our past. We are codependent and have a symbiotic relationship. The beauty of fermentation is that it is easy and can be done in our kitchen. At one point, the bacteria producing lactic acid were declared to be the organisms that humans could use to minimize wasting away their insides (intestines). A Russian-born scientist, Elie Metchnikoff, who studied microbes and their impact on immunity, was convinced that this would help us make longevity attainable.

You must have heard that lactobacillus is found in yogurt (dahi). Many strains, however, do not thrive in our gut. We need to make sure we always have an abundant supply of these. Even though they don't live in our guts, they still perform some important functions and primarily impact our immunity. As explained in the section on leaky gut syndrome, the tight junctions of the intestinal wall give way when dysbiosis occurs. An introduction of the good gut bugs will give you the additional ammunition needed to keep the junctions of the intestinal wall tight. As described by Justin and Erica Sonnenberg, the cells that line our intestines sit side by side and are made up of a network of proteins. The Sonnenbergs call this the grout of these tight junctions.[3] Grout is basically the filling used between two cavities. It's the intestinal wall buffered with grout that keeps the microbiota and the particles of food being digested from crossing into our tissue and bloodstream. Probiotics (which means 'for life'), have been defined by the World Health Organization (WHO) as 'live microorganisms which, when administered in adequate amounts, confer a health benefit on the host'. It can help reinforce the gut barrier by nudging the intestinal cells to produce more protein grout.[4] It also promotes the secretion of mucous that protects our intestinal lining. Probiotics have also been shown to improve other systems beyond the gut, impacting immunity all over.

During the fermentation process, bacteria and yeasts break down proteins into amino acids, fats into fatty acids and complex sugars into simple sugars. Additional compounds are created during this process that benefit the gut and help maintain a healthy ecosystem. Fermentation makes food more absorbable for the body, and enhances the body's ability to assimilate nutrients. For example, in the sauerkraut I make, the vitamin C levels are twenty times more than that present in a regular cabbage. The process is called lacto-fermentation (nothing to do with dairy). Anything that is lacto-fermented is an excellent source of beneficial bacteria or probiotics and enzymes. The process of lacto-fermentation also breaks down phytates, which block mineral absorption. One study found better absorption of iron in people who eat a mix of lacto-fermented vegetables as compared to the same mix of fresh vegetables. The two byproducts of this process are choline and acetylcholine. The beneficial bacteria present in the process of fermentation also serve the role of antibiotics, hindering the growth of harmful microbes/bacteria in the intestine.

Two of the more common bacteria found in fermented foods are lactobacillus and bifidobacteria. These, along with the byproducts of the fermentation process, have the following benefits:

(1) Control of insulin: They tend to alter satiety, and therefore control blood sugar levels.

(2) Controlling inflammation: The influence of the good gut bacteria provided by fermented foods and its impact on maintaining the lining of the intestine, preventing leaky gut or helping in reversing it have been well researched.

(3) Control over leptin and ghrelin: The two hormones that influence hunger are kept under control.

(4) The byproduct choline aids fat metabolism, lowers blood pressure and regulates blood composition.

(5) The byproduct acetylcholine is one of the important neurotransmitters of the body's parasympathetic

nervous system, functionally known to enhance food digestion, decrease heart rate, regulate the internal temperature of the body and lower blood pressure.

(6) The production of SCFAs (that certain good bacteria generate) has been known to control inflammation and help repair the gut, apart from providing energy and extracting calories from your food.

From a macrobiotic perspective, fermentation is the perfect style of food (we say cooking style, as once the salt eats at the vegetable, it's no longer raw; you don't need heat to qualify this as a cooking style) to include in our day-to-day lives. We lead contracted, pressured and yang lives. The energy of quick fermentation with vegetables (by this I mean for 3–10 days)—in an outside environment with salt (yang in its property)—eats into the vegetable in order to break down sugars. The microorganisms produce a bubbling reaction and are alive (so it is live energy, which is yin—upward expansive). The combination of yang and yin elements makes this a perfect style of food to include and bust stress as well, apart from giving us a healthy dose of probiotics. Therefore, it is the most balanced method one could adopt on a daily basis. The overall result is letting your energy slowly move out from deep within, bringing it to the surface of the body. This is very important in a detox.

Jacqueline Fernandez, the Bollywood actress, does all her detox plans with me. I infuse her diet with krauts (pickled cabbage, beetroot or carrots), non-dairy kefirs (more about this later in the book) and kombucha (a drink rich in enzymes).

Types of Fermented Foods (besides Yogurt, Buttermilk and Idli/Dosa)

I have included recipes for you in the Recipe section. However, a lot of these products are coming out under my name this year, so do keep a watch out for them on my website and in retail stores. All fermented foods are superfoods—more beneficial than anything you can do for yourself on a beauty, weight and health level.

Pickling Vegetables

The best way to incorporate fermented foods in your diet from a natural source would be through fermenting vegetables. They are not only packed with fibre, but many phytonutrients ('phyto' means plant in Greek; when plants contain nutrients beneficial to health, we call them phytonutrients) too. This is because they are already cooked with salt and therefore predigested, making nutrients more readily available. When I say 'fermenting vegetables', I mean using a quick-pickling method, unlike the oily, spiced Indian pickles which are cooked for long periods and preserved for a long duration, ultimately killing off the good bacteria. Using saltwater brine or salt, vegetables can be fermented over time durations of one hour, three days or seven days. The ready kraut and pickle or pressed salad (depending upon the duration) are full of probiotics and loaded with enzymes. I have provided recipes for these at the end. Some of them are: sauerkrauts, quick pickles in saltwater brine and *khimchi*.

Kanji

A fermented north Indian drink made with black carrots or beetroots with mustard seeds, kanji takes 3–5 days to ferment. Also referred to as desi wine, it has a distinctly Indian flavour with a hint of mustard. During the process, a lot of polyphenols (known to prevent degenerative diseases) are released, giving it its dark colour. It's generally made in the spring season, which is a good season to do a detox. However, red carrots are usually available in winter and so it is also made at the start of this season.

Rejuvelac

Rejuvelac is a nourishing, energizing fermented tonic. It is a super-sprout drink. The word 'rejuvelac' means 'rejuvenating'. It is a byproduct of the grain-sprouting process. One can use wheat (berries or *gehun*), or any grain like quinoa, amaranth, or any form of millets. Ann Wigmore, a holistic health practitioner fondly called 'the mother of living foods', and the founder of the Hippocrates Health Institute, first brought it to the forefront. Rejuvelac also acts as a natural laxative, and breaks down undigested material in the intestines. The beverage, which should be consumed on empty stomach or between meals, is a bit different as the fermenting process begins from the ground up, like in a kanji. The enzymes to ferment the water are present in the sprouted grain.

Kombucha

Kombucha is a beverage made with tea and sugar, and cultured with something called SCOBY (symbiotic culture of bacteria and yeast), also called the 'mother'. The SCOBY/mother ferments a batch of tea made with some sugar, and the colony of bacteria reproduces (another SCOBY) in seven days. You then get a baby (SCOBY), which you use to ferment the next batch. For kombucha, one needs to obtain the first SCOBY from someone who makes it.

Kefir

Kefir originates in Central Asian Caucasus mountains. It is made with grains and SCOBY. The presence of twenty different strains of bacteria and yeasts, including lactobacilli, gives it a bubbly soda feel and makes it responsible for its 1 per cent alcohol content. It is easy to make if you source the grains. However, all grains require tending to and looking after, and this is the challenge with all cultures. Kefir is known to fight cancer and inflammatory conditions, and regulates immunity. It definitely has been seen to reduce gastrointestinal issues and alleviate allergies during the treatment of my clients (as it reduces the production of cytokines and immunoglobulin E [IgE], which are antibodies produced when the system is attacked by allergens and too much of IgE manifests in allergies, sinusitis, urticaria, dermatitis and food insensitivities). It's a superfood that has also been used to treat hypertension and heart ailments.

Miso

Miso is made by fermenting soybeans and is used in Japanese cooking. You inoculate it with something called *koji,* a Japanese rice-based culture that contains high levels of fungus (the good kind). It's fermented for months or even years, and the result is a paste rich in good microbes. It nourishes your ecosystem like you can't imagine. It sometimes gets a bad rap for having too much sodium, but the level is still much lower than that in table salt. Referred to as a superfood, its nutritional profile is enhanced post fermentation. The fermentation process creates antioxidant compounds, which gives it anticancer properties. You can add it to soups, and like me, to dahls as well; but do not boil it after adding it as this kills off the enzymes (good microbes). It can also be added to chutneys, dips and sauces.

Umeboshi Plum

Besides the dramatic flavour, the Japanese pickled plums have remarkable medicinal qualities. Their powerful acidity has a paradoxical alkalizing effect on the body, preventing fatigue, stimulating digestion and promoting the elimination of toxins and absorption of calcium. In addition, umeboshi is said to help the liver process excess alcohol, restore the skin, help regulate sugar metabolism, prevent or cure anaemia and relieve acute abdominal pain due to gas. Umeboshi is the Far Eastern equivalent of two aspirins and a daily apple. I always have these handy and use them every day—I either just chew on the plum (up to half a day) or use it in the form of chutney (one-fourth teaspoon at a time). It is fantastic to use while travelling, post-hangovers to normalize the system, and on a daily basis if you feel you can handle the sour taste. I have helped avert an asthma attack in a little boy, nine years of age, as we were waiting for the paramedics to arrive. By sucking on the plum, his lung sacks opened up and he could breathe better.

You might question why doctors don't give us probiotic supplements. They only do so when our stomachs are not functioning well. Let me jog your memory back to my introduction wherein I said that your microbiome is different from that of the person next to you. Since all of us have different strains, sometimes it is difficult to orchestrate specific strains of good bacteria that might impact you positively. This is why consuming fermented foods gives you a diverse strain of different bacteria, and a chance of improving and impacting your resident bacteria.

This brings us to the discussion of how we should consume probiotics. As mentioned earlier, fermentation goes back as far as the Rig Veda. Almost all cultures in the world have used some form of fermentation. The truth is Indians have lost the art or distorted it over time. For example, pickling (according to me) is overdone, while it's tasty and adds flavour to our food. Many times, a Gujarati *chunda* has excessive sugar, and even as some of my contemporaries may claim otherwise, sugar is not a superfood. Similarly, north Indians use too much of refined oil and salt to make their pickles and spices. The process of making them is too 'yang'. It can contract you and make you tight. By this I mean that it makes your tissues, muscles and organs tight and will stress you out in the long run if eaten daily over a long period of time. It will also definitely make you crave sweets later (remember yin and yang balance chart). You should consume 1–2 tablespoons of pickles/sauerkraut during each meal and 1 glass of a probiotic beverage (non-dairy) between meals.

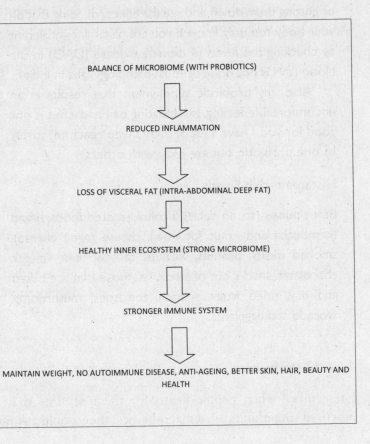

BALANCE OF MICROBIOME (WITH PROBIOTICS)

REDUCED INFLAMMATION

LOSS OF VISCERAL FAT (INTRA-ABDOMINAL DEEP FAT)

HEALTHY INNER ECOSYSTEM (STRONG MICROBIOME)

STRONGER IMMUNE SYSTEM

MAINTAIN WEIGHT, NO AUTOIMMUNE DISEASE, ANTI-AGEING, BETTER SKIN, HAIR, BEAUTY AND HEALTH

> ## Good Gut Bite
>
> ### Histamine Intolerance and Fermented Foods
>
> People who are intolerant of histamine-releasing foods should stay away from fermented foods. Also, if they cause any gas or bloating, you should work on moderating them or cutting them down, and see the effects of doing that on your body. You only know if you are histamine-intolerant by checking the levels of diamine oxidase (DAO) in the blood (this is not done by most pathology labs in India).
>
> Also, any probiotic supplement that results in an uncomfortable feeling, gas, bloating or headaches is not good for you. I have a lot of clients who react negatively to one probiotic, but are okay with others.
>
> ### Histamine-rich Foods
>
> Beans/pulses (so no dahls), alcohol, yeasted foods, bread (kombucha and kraut for now), cheese (aged cheese), smoked meats, peanuts, walnuts, cashew nuts, vinegar, chocolates, snacks out of a box, i.e., those that are baked and dry, dried fruits, spinach, tomatoes, mushrooms, avocado and eggplant.

4. Add Prebiotics

I remember when people heard for the first time that I practised something called macrobiotics, they would ask me if it was the same as probiotics. In 2007, when I began my career, the word 'probiotic' had just taken birth in India. Suddenly, yogurt manufacturers were flaunting it on their labels and Indians were beginning to get familiar with this word. However, no one knew its meaning. Hence, when I said I followed an approach called macrobiotics ('macro' meaning large and 'bios' meaning life—a larger-than-life approach to living), people assumed it was linked to probiotics. While the latter does play a part in macrobiotics, the meanings are completely different.

The role of prebiotics is to provide themselves as fuel for the good microorganisms (probiotic bacteria) to stay healthy and survive. Prebiotics are not living microorganisms, but compounds that are obtained from food. They are complex carbohydrates and an unadulterated version of fibre in foods. They generally only feed the gut bugs and not us. Apart from that, they have numerous benefits: they help you fight insulin resistance and can help with weight loss.

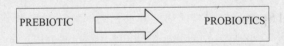

Prebiotic foods like potatoes, sweet potatoes, bananas, onion, garlic, asparagus, apples, avocados, beans, blueberries, chia seeds, garlic, pears, peas, strawberries and chicory—all contain something called inulin, which is high in fibre and low on calories. Many health stores also sell inulin in supplement form, which aids digestion, promotes fullness, reduces cholesterol and, more importantly, provides

SCFAs, the key element needed for energy and protecting our guts from inflammation. All plant-based carbohydrate (fruits and vegetables) fibres are prebiotics.

Good Gut Bite

- Just 8g of prebiotics a day will help absorb minerals, including calcium and magnesium (needed for vitamin D3 and vitamin B12 absorption).
- They help with weight loss, as they make you feel full.
- They reduce glycation, which accelerates ageing and inflammation.
- The cardiovascular burden is reduced as inflammation is controlled.
- They give your good gut bugs a happy feeling.

5. Add Sprouts

By introducing sprouts, you not only take the enzyme (special types of protein that extract vitamins A, B complex, C and E from your food and add essential fatty acids that we do not get in our diet regularly) quotient of your rejuvenate phase up but also make your beans and grain (they can also be sprouted) more digestible. I would recommend adding sprouts for those of you who have a lot of trouble consuming beans and grains in their whole form. Fermenting and sprouting makes it easier to digest these two food groups.

Soaking whole grains and sprouting them removes phytic acid, which prevents absorption of minerals. Sprouting also increases the protein and fibre quotient, as there is less starch in a sprouted bean or grain. To top it off, they have an alkalizing effect on the body, which is also the goal of a detox plan.

In the TCM system, each food corresponds to a season and sprouting comes under the spring season, the perfect time for a detox with the spring equinox on 21 March. Spring brings in new energies and sprouting does just the same when you introduce it in your life. When I need new ideas, thoughts and direction (specifically when I write my books!), I use sprouts a lot in my diet, usually steamed, boiled or sauteed.

6. Add a Bone Soup

In traditional cultures, it was customary to include a bone broth as a part of your diet. All meats were used—beef, chicken, fish or lamb (individually). When I have a client who has gone through severe cycles of chemotherapy and needs energy and supplementation, I recommend a fish broth called *koi-koku* (it's a macrobiotic remedy). It helps the body produce its own collagen, and raise the body's own type 1 collagen found in 90 per cent of all body tissues. Bone soups are excellent to add when healing from a leaky gut, so if you feel your symptoms are severe, adding this to your regimen really helps. Of course this is for non-vegetarians and I will provide the vegetarian equivalent. But there is nothing like a bone soup. Healing compounds

are released in the simmering process from the bones—
collagen, glucosamine (which is taken as a supplement
for joint health), minerals and glutamine, which boost the
immune system. Bovine (cow and buffalo) collagen has type
1 and 2 collagen, beneficial for hair, skin and nails. Because
bone broths are rich in amino acids (proteins), they help heal
the intestinal lining. Besides, it also has L-glutamine, now
touted as a wonder supplement that makes up 35 per cent
of the amino acid nitrogen in your blood. It is an essential
amino acid, known for its help in gaining muscle, enhancing
athletic performance, improving brain health and controlling
blood sugar levels. It is colloquially referred to as the 'band-
aid' for people suffering from leaky gut, prevents diarrhoea
by balancing mucous production, curbs cravings for sugar
and fights cancer. It will also help all the conditions that
come under the umbrella of IBD—ulcerative colitis, Crohn's
disease, diverticulitis, diverticulosis—and others that stem
from inflammation (due to a leaky gut) like joint pain,
rheumatoid arthritis, psoriasis and skin issues. A bone
broth is also known to promote sleep as it has magnesium
and the amino acid glycine. The recommendation is to have
1–2 cups of 250 ml daily.

Good Gut Bite

Foods with L-glutamine: Bone broth, spirulina (sea
algae [good for vegetarians]: see Source List), Chinese
cabbage, tuna, salmon and asparagus.

Shalini, fifty-three, came to me first complaining of severe pain in her joints. Her symptoms revealed she had inflammation. We first went through the common questions I ask someone who is suffering from IBD. She had followed severe crash diets all her life and had very poor digestion, which had led to constipation that she had carried well into her fifties. Weight was not the issue as she was very slim, but she said she had dealt with constipation for as long as she could remember. We changed her diet to one that was basic: whole grains, legumes, vegetables, some superfoods, and a focus on cleaning her up to get her symptoms to abate. She wanted to continue eating eggs (I suspect this came from her dieting days, as most people wanted to keep the diet high on protein by loading up on egg whites). When I told her it was not going to help her stomach, I don't think she was paying attention.

She came back to me in two months saying, 'My body is completely doing its own thing.' She had severe diarrhoea, pain, gas, bloating and stomach cramps after eating meals. She suspected she had SIBO, all thanks to Google! We see this problem everywhere. Those who have even the slightest of issues turn to Google as if it were a doctor.

This time I reiterated that she had a weak microbiome (no balance in her gut microbes) and that this situation over a period of time had led to her leaky gut. Partially digested food had been leaking into her body over a period of time, leading to inflammation and therefore the pain. To help her, I had to bring back her intestinal health and repair her gut lining. This time, I made her do the IgG test, which revealed she was allergic to eggs, something I had been telling her to avoid. She was now serious enough to take on the programme, as she was spending most of her time in the bathroom. Her doctors just put her on more medication, which in a case like this would further weaken her gut. They never explained that an unbalanced microbiome and a leaky gut are the perfect ingredients to give a person an inflammatory response.

I gave her the master detox plan and took her through all the phases of it. I reduced FODMAPs and of course the eggs, and made her follow a simple diet with whole grain (only millet), vegetables, some home-made yogurt (I allowed her this, as she felt it helped her), sauerkraut and another version of a quick pickle, and bone broth with miso paste in it. I told her to keep away from all the triggers outlined in the clean-out phase. She also took a good over-the-counter probiotic, and I stopped all her medication. She has recovered and is still on Phase 3 of the diet as I am writing this book.

This is what she had to say:

'In February 2016, I fell ill. I would have severe bouts of vomiting and diarrhoea with nausea that lasted approximately eight hours, every ten days. I saw my general practitioner and a gastroenterologist, and tried the usual cocktail of medicines, and these only made me sicker. When I was asked to do invasive tests to determine why I was not healing, I switched tracks and approached Shonali for help.

'Her advice was to start with a food intolerance test, avoid food that didn't suit me and then start eating right to repair my gut.

'She added prebiotics, probiotics in the form of fermented foods, bone broths and whole grains like brown rice, and followed a limited-fibre approach. Then she slowly increased the fibre in my diet and eliminated sugar. It took a few months (six), as she had predicted, but I am now completely well.

'Her advice on how to eat was invaluable, but her steady reassurance through the process that I would heal completely was equally important as well.'

What Should You Expect from Phase 3?

Phase 3 is the whole shebang as I mentioned. This is where you will see some major shifts taking place. You will lose weight (especially water weight), your energy levels will be high, bowel movements will be better, skin will clear up, you will feel less bloated, look great, be happier and calmer. Use it to also clear up negative feelings, emotions and grudges you may be holding on to. Detoxes stir up all the toxic substances in your liver and bring it to the surface. That's why it is recommended to start them in spring (which, according to the TCM doctrine, is the season of the liver). The liver also houses anger as an emotion, so detoxes help you shake out the anger as well.

9

TOP IT UP

Phase 4: This Phase Is to Be Added in the Last Week of the Rejuvenate Phase and Should Become a Mainstay in Your Life

'Antioxidant' is the buzzword these days, known varyingly as 'saviours' or 'gatekeepers' of our immunity, superfoods and oxygenators for our cells. They add another dimension to our existence. They improve health, mind, body and performance levels, and add to our beauty, glow and happiness levels. Antioxidants are a class of molecules that are capable of inhibiting the oxidation generated by another class of molecules. Your body's natural antioxidant capacity declines with age, so it's good to keep it coming from all sources.

Let's get into this more closely. What is a free radical? It is a reactive substance that is basically a molecule with an odd number of electrons, looking to balance itself by stealing from the ones around it. If there are too many floating around, they constantly try to balance themselves and affect your cells. This is when free-radical damage happens; they interact with tissues, causing damage. It's a big reason for our ageing. Essentially, this free-radical damage is similar to the process by which rust is formed. This happens to the tissues in your body by a process called oxidation. The Ayurvedic theory on build-up of ama is basically the same as free-radical damage. We can protect ourselves using a diet that is optimized with minimal sugars and plenty of vegetables. Sugar generates more free radicals, and vegetables decrease the damage from it. Antioxidants give it an electron to rebalance itself, so they don't steal from your cells. If you don't supply yourself with adequate antioxidants, they will not thwart the production of free radicals, and it will accelerate the ageing process.

It's important to understand antioxidants, since a lot of people ask me how to up the level of these in the body. Antioxidants are soluble in lipids (fat) or water, both of which are important for cells. The cell membranes are made up of fat, while the cells themselves have water. Free radicals do not discern which cells they will attack, so you need to have both types of antioxidants to ensure the cells outlive this destruction by free radicals. This means you basically need a wide variety of them.

Topping up the perfect master detox diet is like a director wrapping up the last scene or a chef like me adding the final garnish to your dish.

In this phase, I will outline all the antioxidants via foods and supplements that you could use to top up your detox.

This will give you a magnified version of your cleanse. However, these foods are recommended when you finish with the previous phase, and go on to a slightly more routine way of eating.

Sounds exciting? Yes, it is. A lot of people ask me the mystery behind my healthy skin glow. When I think about it, I realize I have taken this for granted. I have eaten well (healthy) pretty much from my twenties, though you may say genes have a lot to do with it. (Yes, my mom and dad had great skin, so did my grandparents. My dad's family hailed from Peshawar and there was definitely some mixing in that gene pool. Sabherwals can trace their lineage to King Porus. Mom's family, on the other hand, hailed from Sialkot [Pakistan], and my maternal grandmother had great skin.) While this may have been 20 per cent of the cause, 80 per cent of what I am has been the result of my eating habits from my twenties.

My Diet

The foods outlined in the clean-out phase have been out of my life since my late twenties. I am not a meat eater, but I do have fish, and I do have at least five types of fermented products in a day. I stick to organic whole grains: mainly brown rice and foxtail millet (cheena), lots of vegetables (specifically lots of leafy greens), legumes, fruit and herbal teas. Every diet needs to be supplemented with magic bullets of energy and antioxidants. Only then do they show results. Just having these in your life, without a solid diet, will not work. Like I say, every decade determines the next, and that's been the case with my age, skin, energy levels and overall health; it just keeps getting better and better. Some of the top-ups will overlap, which means one food may give you multiple benefits.

> ### Good Gut Bite
>
> Sweet potatoes are among the top ten foods that defy ageing. Rich in beta carotene, which the body converts to vitamin A, they keep your skin smooth and wrinkle-free. It is high in MAC fibre (one sweet potato contains 4g of fibre), rich in iron and calcium and has a low glycaemic index. It strengthens the spleen and pancreas; promotes qi energy; removes toxins; builds the kidneys; and is useful to treat diarrhoea. It houses powerful antioxidants that work in the body to remove free radicals. Sweet potato is a good food for diabetics, because it helps stabilize blood sugar levels and balances the sodium/potassium ratio of the body. It is also rich in serotonin, which is a mood booster. I recommend this to all my clients with depression, Asperger's syndrome and mind disorders.

Top It Up with Glutathione (Glutamylcysteinylglycine or GSH, Comprising Three Key Amino Acids)

A non-enzymatic antioxidant, GSH is known not only to help the cells but is also the single most important aspect of every cell, i.e., every cell of your body produces it. It also helps enhance the effects of other antioxidants and fruits and vegetables you eat daily. Inflammation is a common cause for inadequate oxygenation of the blood in the tissues; this is why GSH is crucial. It not only helps with the immune function but also increases the body's T-cells, which fight cancer. The body's ability to produce it declines as you age, but certain foods do help. Raw foods usually have more GSH. Curcumin, garlic, avocado, asparagus, spinach, arugula, kale, mustard greens (*sarson*), potatoes, melons, peaches, strawberries, cabbage, broccoli, cauliflower, Brussels sprouts, radish, turnip (shalgam), cinnamon and cardamom are the main foods with GSH. Beets, lentils, chickpeas, kidney beans and black beans keep up the production of GSH. Including food with vitamin C, such as oranges, red pepper, green peppers, guava, strawberries, grapefruit and kiwi, and vitamin E, such as sweet potato, seeds, almonds, wheat germ, red pumpkin, avocado and olive oil, also helps produce GSH.

Top It Up with Alpha Lipoic Acid (ALA)

Made naturally in our bodies, ALA is also found in many plant foods. It is positively correlated with controlling insulin sensitivity, protecting skin collagen (specifically skin damaged by over-abuse of sugar in the diet), cleaning up the liver, absorbing free radicals, slowing down the ageing process and fighting inflammation. It has been known to work as a team with B vitamins, turning all the macronutrients from food into energy that is utilized by the body. Foods with ALA are spinach, broccoli, yams, potatoes, carrots, beetroot, rice bran and brewer's yeast. In supplement format, 300–600 mg is recommended.

Top It Up with Coenzyme Q10 (CoQ10)

Known to many to actually support heart health, CoQ10 helps produce more energy for your cells. The body makes it in the liver. It is termed as a 'universal antioxidant' and is definitely used for anti-ageing. It is found in wines, grapes, certain fruits, vegetables like spinach, broccoli and cauliflower, and in mackerel, sardines, beef, poultry, nuts, seeds and oils. In supplement form, 30–200 mg a day is recommended, for people between the ages of 40–60 and of good health.

Top It Up with Coloured Vegetables and Fruits (Carotenoids)

Think colours (glow givers) when you think of antioxidants from your foods: Carrots, tomatoes (lycopene), red, green and yellow peppers, red pumpkin (lal kaddu/bhopla), apples, spring onions, watermelons, mangoes, papayas, peaches, apricots, red/black berries, corns, bananas, leafy greens (will help you fight facial lines), okra (bhindi), green beans, kale, cabbage and avocado. Carotenoids help convert to vitamin A, which is vital for tissue repair. Cruciferous vegetables like cauliflower, broccoli and Brussels sprouts will clean up the excess of hormones.

Top It Up with Vitamin C

Mainly known in the beauty industry for collagen regeneration, vitamin C is a major player in the fight against inflammation. It helps with tissues, tendons, bones and blood vessel repair. It also helps the body synthesize calcium. Foods high in vitamin C are: citrus fruits, guava, melons, *amalaki* (*amla*), dark leafy greens, papaya, bell peppers, broccoli, strawberries, pineapples, oranges, kiwi, cantaloupe, cauliflower, coriander (*dhaniya*), chives, thyme, basil and parsley.

Top It Up with B Vitamins

B vitamins help fight any gut inflammation issue. Important ones are vitamin B6, B9 and vitamin B12 (you get vitamin B12 in abundant supply from all fermented foods). Adding whole grains to your diet also takes up the B vitamin profile. Remember, biotin—the supplement for hair, skin and nails—supports adrenal function and is basically the vitamin B7 found in nut butters, nuts, mushrooms, salmon, dark berries, soybeans, barley, brewer's yeast and whole grains. Get more from the B vitamins by adding lentils, nuts, yogurt (if you eat dairy), tuna, turkey, potato, sweet potato, banana, sunflower seeds, spinach, avocado and kidney beans.

Top It Up with Turmeric

I eat a raw turmeric (*kachcha* haldi) pickle daily (see recipe). I buy it when it's in season or just use the powder.

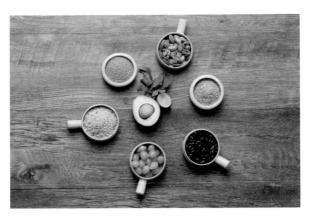

The detox diet food groups

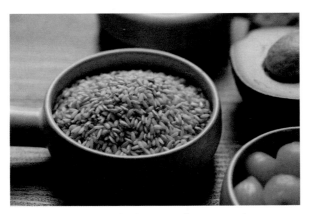

MAC 1: Whole grains (brown rice)

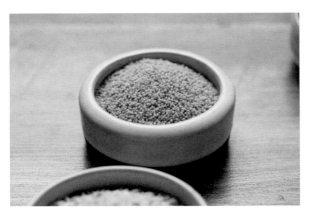

MAC 1: Foxtail millet

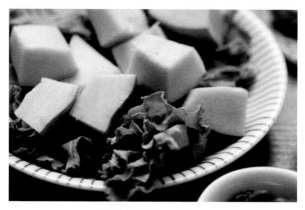

MAC 2: Vegetables

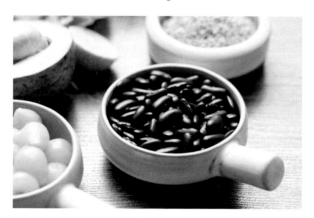

MAC 4: Legumes

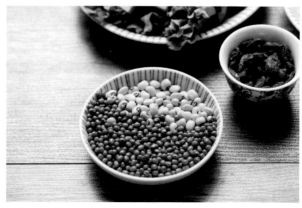

MAC 4: Yin-yang beans

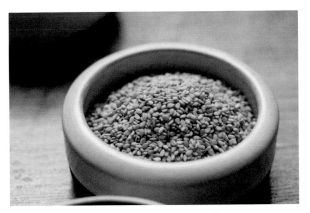

MAC 5: Seeds (sesame)

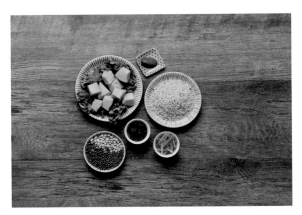

Detox diet foods and proportions

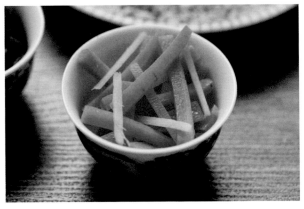

Pickled carrots and ginger

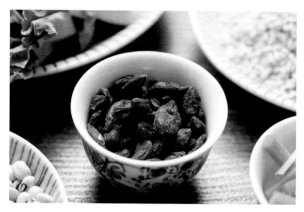

Superfood goji berries

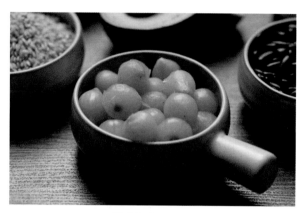

Pickled onions

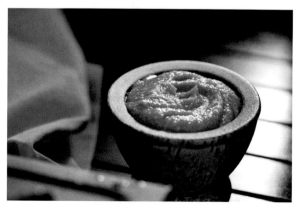

Fermented food: Miso paste

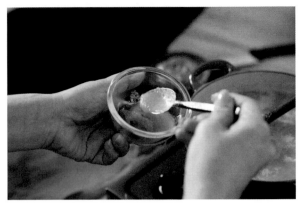

Mixing miso paste in soup

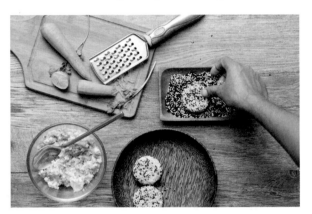

Brown-rice croquettes

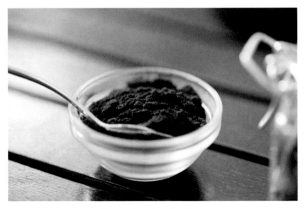

Superfood spirulina

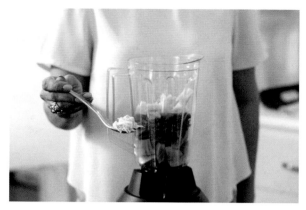

Mixing sauerkraut in a smoothie

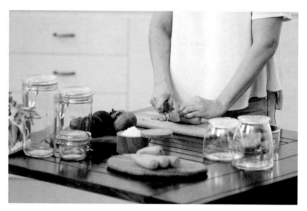

Chopping from *hara*, the second chakra

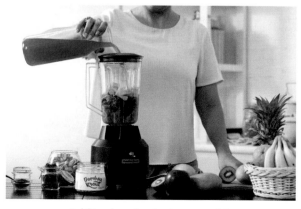

Adding kombucha to smoothie

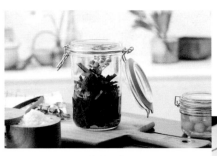

Fermented foods: Beetroot
kraut and onion pickle

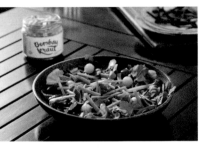

Carrot kraut added to salad

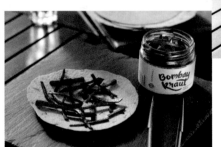

Beetroot kraut on khakra

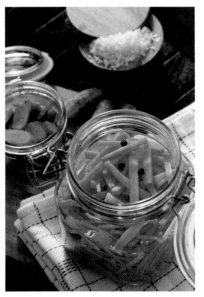

Yin-yang carrot pickle

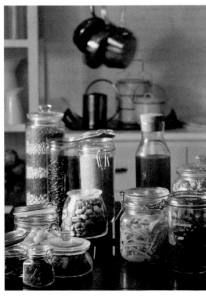

Major food groups to build gut bacteria

Sauerkraut Procedure

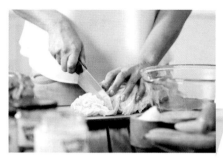

1. Chop the cabbage

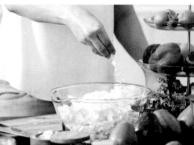

2. Add sea or rock salt

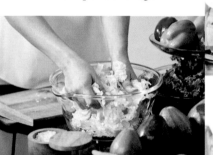

3. Rub the sea salt into the cabbage

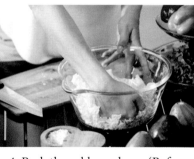

4. Pack the cabbage down (Refer to the diagram on page 278 on how to ferment the sauerkraut before bottling)

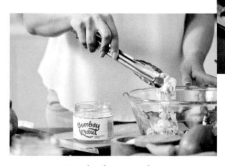

5. Bottle the sauerkraut

Its primary active agent, curcumin, has been known to have anti-inflammatory properties. It works with all the ailments listed earlier under IBD and inflammation. Relevant to the central theory of this book and aiding us in fighting against the bad microbes, and creating good biodiversity in our guts, curcumin decreases the harmful seepage of toxins from the gut to the human body, and helps calm the immune response. It has been known to help with the fight against generation of more fat storage in the cells and decreasing body weight, with a good diet in place. It also elevates tryptophan and serotonin, which help lower appetite. Remember the connection between chronic inflammation and weight gain? When you are in this state, you are deficient in adiponectin (a protein involved in regulation of glucose and fatty acid breakdown). Curcumin increases adiponectin, impacting insulin levels. It has been known to have blood-thinning qualities, and positively impacts lipid metabolism, helping to lower bad cholesterol. The West is now selling it in capsules, as they do not use it on an everyday basis.

Top It Up with Bitter Foods (the Liver Loves It)

According to TCM, bitter and sour foods reduce excesses in liver. In a detox, we are supposed to cleanse the liver. Perhaps the most powerful common remedy for quickly removing liver stagnation and indigestion is vinegar. Choose unrefined apple cider vinegar (you can add honey to increase effectiveness). It cools down the heat in the liver caused by overconsumption of rich foods. The property that accompanies a bitter flavour is yin (cooling), causing the energy of the body to descend. Bitter flavours help lower a fever. It also helps the heart by cleaning the arteries of damp mucoid deposits of cholesterol and fats, in turn lowering blood pressure. The kidney and lungs are vitalized by the bitter flavours, which are also superb for removing mucous/heat conditions in the lungs, signified by phlegm discharges. Bitter foods you should use are arugula leaves, celery, romaine lettuce, alfalfa, dark chocolate, sauerkraut, turmeric, fenugreek, bitter gourd (*karela*), *baunphal* (dandelion), grapefruit, olive, bitter melon, bitter and sweet asparagus, amaranth (*rajgeera*), papaya, curry leaves, mustard seeds, bay leaves (*tej patta*), neem leaves, licorice root (*mulhathi*), stevia and some vinegars.

Top It Up with Coconut Oil (Cold-Pressed) for Medium-Chain Fatty Acids (MCFAs)

Coconut oil is high on MCFAs. While most oils take longer time to digest, coconut oil is one of the best saturated fats (apart from ghee) that hits the liver and bypasses the digestive system, providing instant energy. Besides this ability, it is antimicrobial and antifungal, and does not get stored as fat in the body. It has anti-inflammatory compounds, is also known to be a pain reliever and kills off *Helicobacter pylori*, which could impact stomach ailments. Lauric acid, which is one of its components, is known to reduce candida, fight negative bacteria and maintain the inner ecosystem. Coconut oil also helps digestion and makes it easier to absorb magnesium, calcium and fat-soluble vitamins. For example, if consumed with omega-3 fatty acids, it can have a more positive effect on the body. It is positively correlated with weight loss, as it increases the body's metabolism, causing a thermogenic effect known to decrease appetite and burn fat. Here is how you can top it up with coconut oil:

Twenty minutes before each meal, take some cold-pressed coconut oil as an infusion in warm water or herbal teas.

(1) If you weigh 40–60kg, take 1 tablespoon before each meal, for a total of 3 tablespoons a day.
(2) If you weigh 60–80kg, take 1½ tablespoons before each meal, for a total of 4½ tablespoons a day.
(3) If you weigh over 80kg, take 2 tablespoons before each meal, for a total of 6 tablespoons a day.

Note: On any diet, you must eat half your fats from the good saturated fats or you will have trouble keeping energy between meals, which will cause carbohydrate cravings. You must get 2–6g of omega-3 and the rest can be omega-9. Also, you can add 1 teaspoon of cod liver or flax oil before breakfast if you include omega-3 daily.[1]

Top It Up with Ghee

Ghee features everywhere in Indian cooking. And there's a good reason for it. According to the Ayurvedic tradition, it enhances *ojas* (Sanskrit for vigour), an essence that governs the tissues in the body and balances hormones. Apart from that, ghee has a very high smoke point and doesn't burn easily during cooking. It has more stable saturated bonds and so is less likely to form dangerous free radicals when cooking, which is what usually causes free-radical damage in Indians. During the process of clarifying milk to obtain ghee, proteins are removed and it becomes lactose-free, thereby increasing its nutritional value. Ghee has been known to fight inflammation, have positive effects on insulin sensitivity and intestinal permeability, maintain gut-barrier integrity, increase absorption of water in the gut and hence prevent leaky gut syndrome. Ghee is an antioxidant in this respect. My recommendation is 1 tablespoon a day.

Top It Up with Ashwagandha

Considered one of the most powerful Ayurvedic herbs, ashwagandha means 'the smell of a horse' in Sanskrit. This actually translates to the vigour and vitality of a horse. It has properties that calm you mentally, and restore and rejuvenate you. Some of its benefits are stress reduction, better immunity, reduced anxiety, enhanced libido and stabilization of blood sugars. It is especially helpful for people with hypo- or hyperthyroidism.

Top It Up with Shilajit

I remember I got introduced to shilajit when my father was diagnosed with cancer, and we went to meet Mona Schwartz to learn macrobiotics to help him at the time. She brought out this rock-like black mineral from her refrigerator, and said we should start him on it right away. It is known as the 'destroyer of weaknesses' and the 'conquerer of mountains'. Found in large concentrations in the Himalayas, shilajit contains over fifty different trace minerals. Since our Indian diets lack the necessary trace minerals, it's recommended that we incorporate it in our diet. It prevents cell damage and oxidative damage due to free-radical overload. Therefore, it helps slow down the ageing process, enhances libido and provides many cofactors that help enzyme action.

Top It Up with Sea Vegetables

One sea vegetable I mentioned before is kombu, which is available in India (see Source List). A source of abundant trace minerals, with a high content of calcium and iron, it also has the highest iodine content among all seaweeds. It is definitely an antioxidant and is known to be detoxifying and alkalizing, and it purifies the blood. Another sea vegetable now available in India is spirulina, rich in chlorophyll, which mimics the molecular structure of haemoglobin (red blood cells) and helps build good, strong blood. All sea vegetables are prebiotic and beneficial for the microbes in your gut. They all have amazing detoxification properties.

Top It Up with Shiitake Mushrooms

Shiitake mushrooms are now available widely in our Indian market. Since ancient times, shiitake has been highly valued as both food and medicine. Wu Ri, a famous physician from the Chinese Ming dynasty, wrote extensively about this mushroom, noting its ability to increase energy, cure colds and eliminate worms. Traditional Chinese physicians knew the power of the dark, meaty, capped, forest mushroom to activate qi or life force and promote longevity.

Dried shiitake contains 25 per cent protein, and all eight essential amino acids are present in a ratio similar to the 'ideal' protein for human nutrition. Shiitake is rich in leucine and lysine, which are deficient in many grains. It has high levels of glutamic acid, which is considered to be a 'brain food' due to its ability to stimulate neurotransmitter activity as well as its ability to transport potassium to the brain. It is rich in vitamin B12 (not available in vegetables, only synthesized by bacteria and fungi), riboflavin, niacin, copper, selenium, zinc, dietary fibre and enzymes. It also contains ergosterol, which converts to vitamin D. Shiitake mushrooms also contain an active compound called lentinan, a polysaccharide that strengthens the response of our immune system.

Top It Up with Vinegar

The first advocate of drinking vinegar was Hippocrates, the father of modern medicine. This doesn't mean that you go to your local bania and get any vinegar that is available off the shelf. What you need is unpasteurized vinegar that contains a number of vitamins and minerals. It is known to have as many as fifty nutrients and also the benefits of the fruit it comes from. Nowadays people are crazy about apple cider vinegar and consume it aimlessly without even knowing what it is actually doing for them and why. North

African women have used it for very long as a weight-loss agent. On a detox, I would suggest to use it for its probiotic benefits, as it improves inclusion of good microbes in your gut. Add it to salad dressings or chug it; I prefer the former.

Here are two handy tips:

(1) Mix 1 tablespoon with 8 ounces or 2 teaspoons with 16 ounces of water and consume.
(2) Have it before a meal if you suffer from heartburn, and at any other time of the day for those who are using it as a probiotic.

Note: It may activate your stomach to have a bowel movement, so make sure you are near a bathroom if you are introducing it in your life for the first time.

Top It Up with Magnesium (Citrate or Glycinate)

A magnesium supplement can encourage bowel movements and calm down the gut as well. Having 200–800 mg per day at bedtime is a good start.

10

OXYGENATE

'We can look at oxygen deficiency or oxygen starvation as the single greatest cause of all disease.'
—Stephen Levine[1]

In this section, I walk you through the ways to enhance your life through your attitude, lifestyle habits and add-ons to help sustain a healthier life. The first steps of laying the groundwork for maintaining a balance in life has begun. If you have implemented the first four phases of the diet, you will find a sea change in how your gut responds and what you look like on the outside, which mirrors your insides. My principles in life have always been to find ways to complement my healthy eating habits with simple, sustainable lifestyle 'add-ons' that help me take my health to the next level. This could range from exercising to breathing (pranayam). Here are a few habits that I have cultivated to bring in more 'oxygen' into my life and allow my cells to breathe and restore.

Of all the nutrients, oxygen is the most essential. Symbolized by the letter 'O', it has a more fundamental nutritional role than vitamins, minerals or any other. Everyone knows that human life ends within a few minutes without oxygen, but not enough people are aware of the often chronic oxygen starvation of their own tissues and cells. Your cells need oxygen to live. Toxins block the cellular oxygen respiration mechanism.

The body is 75 per cent water, and oxygen accounts for nearly 90 per cent of the weight of water. It may be considered a yang force. Without it, the fuel in the body cannot burn for energy or heat. The red blood cells carry it to every part of the body; insufficient levels of oxygen can result in anaemia. The qi of Chinese medicine (or prana of Ayurvedic medicine) has a direct relationship to oxygen; in fact, qi is sometimes translated as 'breath'. Modern perspectives on oxygen give it several functions identical to those of qi: it energizes the body, clears obstructions and overcomes stagnancy. When one is lacking in oxygen, one feels heavy, depressed and devoid of vitality. It is also needed for vitamin C utilization, to retard collagen breakdown and to prevent premature ageing. A person with adequate cellular oxygen has a greater capacity to be outgoing (yang) and socially successful; people are attracted to the charisma that comes from abundant oxygen.

The brain and the heart utilize most of the oxygen we inhale; the liver also requires it to rebuild its cells. Oxygen therapy greatly benefits alcoholics and others who have damaged their livers and brain functions. Once sufficient oxygen is in the system, one feels charged with life and is usually no longer attracted to intoxicants.

Another important role of oxygen is that of a purifier, helping eliminate wastes in the body. It destroys germs, viruses, amoebas, parasites, fungi and yeasts (essentially, it is the best to get rid of all the bad microorganisms in the gut) and resolves pathogenic moisture (dampness) in the form of oedema, mucus, cysts, tumours and arterial plaque. To understand its power, consider a commonly observed form of oxygen, ozone (O_3). It is recognized worldwide for purifying water by eliminating chemicals and pesticides through oxidation and by destroying all microorganisms. It is a substantially better purifier than chlorine and additionally has none of the side effects.

Generally, more oxygen is needed by those who are overweight, sluggish, or who have candidiasis, oedema, heart disease, IBD, autoimmune disorders, chronic fatigue syndrome, viral/timorous infections (e.g., cancer, multiple sclerosis, rheumatoid arthritis, AIDS) or a compromised immune system.[2]

Oxygenation

The following practices outlined in this section will help to increase and distribute oxygen in the body.

Oxygenation via Pranayams

Most people don't know that I am a certified Yogalates teacher. It is a fitness routine that combines yoga and Pilates, developed by a lady called Louise Solomon in Byron Bay, Australia. Here, we teach yogic pranayams, which we practise throughout our mat-work class. This is designed to enrich you with oxygen, while getting a workout as well.

Belly Breathing/Full Diaphragmatic Breathing

Technique

(1) Lie flat on the floor on a yoga mat.
(2) Bring legs in towards buttocks at a 90-degree angle at knees.
(3) Place a cushion under your head for comfort.
(4) Place one hand on the abdomen and the other on the side of the chest.
(5) Inhale smoothly and evenly through the nose without strain.
(6) Feel the abdomen gently rising under the lower hand (like a balloon inflating). There should be little or no movement under the upper hand.
(7) Exhale smoothly, feeling the abdomen sink gently (like a deflating balloon).
(8) Sense or visualize the rhythm of the diaphragm massaging the internal organs.

Benefits

(1) Activates the parasympathetic nervous system.
(2) Relaxes the body.
(3) Teaches the body to maximize the use of the diaphragm, which is responsible for 70–80 per cent of natural breathing.
(4) Increases lung capacity.

(5) Enhances the quality of sleep (should be done at bedtime).
(6) Focuses the mind, assisting in relaxing the body in times of high anxiety and stress.
(7) May assist in menstrual cramping and digestive disorders.

Contraindications

Belly breathing is a very simple and safe practice, but it is not advised in the case of the contraindications listed below:

(1) Dizziness or pressure behind the ears.
(2) Acute hernias.
(3) Respiratory disorders.
(4) Recent abdominal surgery.
(5) Heavy menstruation.

Ujjayi Breath

Ujjayi (pronounced *oo-jai*) is also referred to as 'the ocean breath' or 'the victorious breath'—it increases oxygenation and builds internal body heat.

Technique

(1) Seal lips and start breathing in and out through the nose.
(2) Inhale through the nose slowly, and while exhaling, constrict the muscles at the back of the throat.

(3) It is performed by contracting the glottis in the throat, which happens when we tuck the chin into the throat.

(4) It feels like deep breathing, involving the throat, like gentle snoring or the sound of a baby sleeping.

Benefits

(1) Has a serene effect on the nervous system, calming the mind.

(2) Reduces heartbeat and therefore helps those with high blood pressure.

(3) Detoxifies mind and body.

(4) Increases oxygen in the blood.

Contraindications

Ujjayi Breath is a very simple and safe practice, but it is not advised in the case of the contraindications listed below:

(1) Anxiety.

(2) Low blood pressure.

(3) Neck pain.

(4) Throat-constriction issues.

(5) If on an immunosuppressant.

(6) Blocked nose.

Oxygenation via Movement

Whatever kind of movement you do, be it swimming, cycling, working out or hiking—it will increase oxygen and endorphins, the two things you could use on a detox for sure. Movement increases circulation, so definitely plan on doing something to increase it.

Oxygenation via Massage

Massage is integral, especially a lymphatic drainage massage. You have twice as much lymph fluid as blood in your body. Lymph is a fine network of tissues and organs that gets rid of the toxic build-up of wastes in your body; it supports the lymph fluid, which contains white blood cells—the soldiers of your body. So supporting them is essential. Digestive disorders and stress are major reasons why a lymph system might be congested. I get two massages done a week, and follow the Kerala style of Ayurveda. You should pick one that suits you and stick to it as a routine; even once a week is enough.

Oxygenation via a Body Scrub

Your skin is the largest organ after your microbiome. Each square centimetre of skin may have up to 600 sweat glands, twenty blood vessels, 6000 melanocytes and over a thousand nerve endings. Among the many functions of the skin are protection, sensation, heat regulation, excretion of sweat, and water resistance (to keep nutrients from washing out of your body). Your skin is connected to your capillaries, main arteries, veins and, through them, your circulatory system, which is discharging toxins 24/7.

Foods such as saturated fats from dairy and meats, and eggs, clog up your skin, preventing the passage and elimination of both moisture and oil through your pores. If excess fat is sent back into your circulatory system through the blood vessels, detoxification becomes harder.

Body scrubs help to activate blood circulation and the lymphatic system as well. They exfoliate your skin, sloughing off dead skin cells, rubbing away hard, flaky skin and also pulling out the discharge that is released through the pores (i.e., toxins). A body scrub can be very invigorating, as it improves blood circulation, fights cellulite and improves skin tone. It is one anti-ageing secret which I use daily.

Good Gut Bite

How to Do a Body Scrub

Take a small tub and fill it with hot water (as hot as you can bear); or do it with hot running water under the shower. Take a cotton washcloth. Dip the cloth in the hot water and squeeze the excess water. Rub skin vigorously, wetting the cloth once you finish one area of your body. So, for example, if you are done with one arm, wet the cloth again and do the other arm. Do it on every part of the body (buttocks, back of the neck, behind the ears, between the toes). Don't forget the face. Focus on the joints as maximum discharge gathers around the joints).

Benefits

(1)   Makes you feel lighter.
(2)   Makes you more energetic.
(3)   Makes you sleep better.
(4)   Brings improvement in muscle tone.
(5)   Makes your skin glow.
(6)   Brings spring in your gait.

The Good Gut Poses (Asanas)

I am enumerating the good gut poses. I recommend that you get a yoga teacher to teach them to you. These poses are better learnt under supervision. I am, however, giving you pictures as a reference.

Triangle Pose (*Trikonasana*)

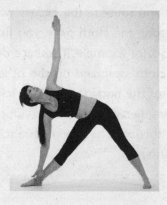

Revolved Triangle Pose (*Parivritta* Trikonasana)

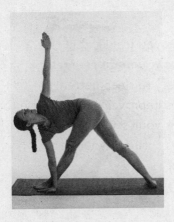

Cat to Cow (*Marjaryasana Bitilasana*)

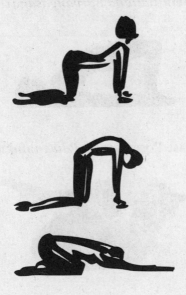

Downward-Facing Dog (*Adho Mukha Svanasana*)

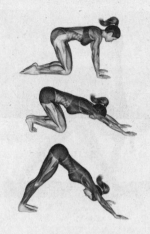

Bridge Pose (*Setu Bandha Sarvangasana*)

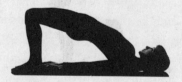

Half Gas Release Pose (*Ardha Pawanmuktasana*)

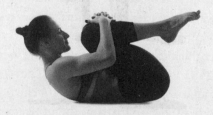

Supine Twist (*Supta Matsyendrasana*)

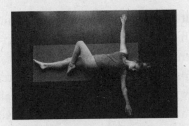

Other Methods of Oxygenation

Here are some other tips on increasing the oxygen content in our life:

(1) Have plenty of plants around you. They definitely help in increasing the oxygen uptake.

(2) Open your windows, let the fresh air come in (reminds me of my school teacher who'd say, 'let the "climate" come in'). This will help you absorb all that good, fresh oxygen.

(3) Practise meditation. Just focusing on the incoming and outgoing breath will increase the oxygen uptake.

(4) Eat greens rich in chlorophyll, which has magnesium at its centre. This changes to iron that transports oxygenated blood everywhere in our body.

(5) Massage increases circulation, which results in more oxygen being carried to our cells.

(6) Water purification units using ozone increase oxygen levels in the water, so check if you have one of those.

(7) Staying hydrated is important for the transportation of body fluids, apart from the utilization of oxygen.

Develop Some Lifestyle Traits

(1) Be in gratitude: Having immense amount of gratitude for everything in your life not only changes your health (mental and psychological) but also improves relationships, makes you sleep better, keeps you optimistic, increases self-esteem, makes you less egocentric and self-absorbed, more relaxed and most of all a kinder person. We are here for a divine purpose, which is larger than your small problems and issues. If you can be connected to that one thought, you will 'defocus' from everything else.

(2) Be resilient: In his book *The Gut Balance Revolution*, Gerard Mullin talks about being resilient. He cites Dr Mehmet Oz, who says being resilient is the key to reversing the ageing process.[3] Resilience is defined as the ability to bounce back from an illness, challenge or life event without developing a maladaptive chronic stress response. The more resilient you are, the less physically or emotionally affected you will be by life's stressors. This will enable you to bounce back when a setback occurs. As the first noble truth stated in Buddhism states: 'Life is suffering, to live you must suffer. It is impossible to live without experiencing some kind of suffering.' This is not to sound too pessimistic; however, this is actually the truth. So why not cultivate some resiliency.

I believe I have this one trait in such abundance that I can write books on the subject. I have always managed to face reality, no matter how harsh, and found greater meaning in my down times. I have also been able to make do with what I have at hand, and constantly innovate and improvise. I never say 'why me', but always say 'why not?'

(3) Examine emotional baggage: Start addressing all emotional traumas; use whatever it takes to sort them out. Whether it means chanting, joining a support group, finding what makes you tick, writing a journal or seeking psychotherapy—catharsis is something one needs to move on.

(4) Declutter your life: This would mean people, things and situations that do not define you any more. Surround yourself with positive people and things. This doesn't mean you start collecting things again; keep it minimalistic.

(5) Set boundaries: We tend to be over-nurturers, I know I am, but we need to know our own limitations and accept them. So set boundaries, even with your kids, pets, husband, in-laws, workers and boss. Know that there is only so much that you can do.

(6) Use bodywork therapies: This includes acupuncture, acupressure and craniosacral therapy (see Source List). All these bodywork therapies aim to balance you. They go beyond medicines and tap into your emotional state.

(7) Take ten minutes a day to connect with the 'source': You can call this source of energy the divine, prana or qi—whatever you want. But if meditation is a way to connect with the source, keeping aside even ten minutes a day to do so would help. Sit blank, pray, walk alone, dance, sing, do anything, but be grateful for your life.

(8) Meditate: Meditation has been a part of Indian cultural heritage. 'Being present' or 'living in the now' is key to this. Now the same concept has been given a makeover in the West and called 'mindfulness'. You have to be aware only of what's going on in the present. A simple way to implement it could be through the mindfulness of your meals—begin eating with no distractions; just you and your food. Give your food your 100 per cent, which means focus on chewing, the flavours, how it tastes, its texture, and respecting that it's present in your life.

(9) Add laughter: Be it visiting a comedy club, watching a funny movie, reading something funny or simply getting together with friends and enjoying, just laugh.

(10) Look at your life from different 'realms': Sometimes, creating a 'shift' in the way you look at stuff in your life really helps. This also comes from knowing deep inside you that you are connected to something much larger than just the mundane stuff in life. We often need to shift our consciousness and come from higher realms (see picture). If we are stuck in anger, fear and desire, and feel victimized, we are only functioning on a physical realm. However, we must strive to come from a 'spiritual' realm—that of unconditional love, acceptance, wisdom and reason. It is important to know our soul has its own destiny, that we are on this planet for a purpose, and that the drama that unfolds is a part of the plan. I have to thank my friend Dilshad Pastakia for introducing me to this way of thinking.

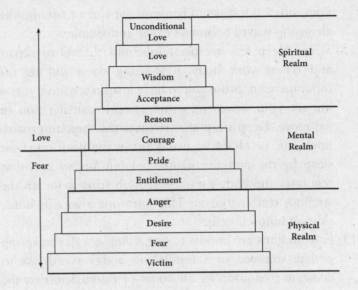

(11) Develop some lifestyle habits of eating: When I deal with my clients, I see that a lot of them don't just eat unhealthy but also maintain unhealthy lifestyle habits—by eating their meals and sleeping at odd hours. Good habits are also very important in keeping your body's energy clock in harmony; each organ has its own timing, and adhering to these helps them do their job. Otherwise, it can throw your gut off and develop unhealthy gut microbes. The gut will undergo some contractions during what Gerard Mullin calls a 'cleansing wave'.[4] This is when bad bugs don't take seat in your gut and digestion happens. When you eat on time, the cleansing wave is called into action to drown out the bad bugs, and shift remainders of the food to

your small intestine. When you eat out of timing, the cleansing waves become weaker and smaller.

(12) Sleep: Sleep has a crucial job, and that is to repair and renew your body. Restricting sleep will set off inflammation, cause you to have insulin sensitivity, and impact your neuroendocrine system, causing you to eat more. Deep sleep also releases the 'human growth hormone' or HGH, squirted out in the deep stages of sleep by the pituitary gland. It is an amino acid that regulates the body's muscle growth (this is for all the strength training guys). This hormone also aids bone, skin and muscle cells.

(13) Fast: Indians are known to fast. Choose a day in spring or late summer, or a festival, or a day you'd like to dedicate to a god. We all know of *Paryushan* that the Jains are famous for. It is a method of fasting to cleanse their soul. It's not only done with a view to cleansing the body, but also the higher self. It is a time to reflect on your life in the year gone by and practise forgiveness. I respect this community for its practices, and this is one thing that many Jains follow once a year. Fasting has immense benefits: it reduces insulin sensitivity, helps manage stress, reduces free radical damage and ends up supporting the microbiota, also imparting longevity. In my Ayurvedic cleanse, there is a treatment called *Rasayanan* ('rasa' means gold; it is the Ayurvedic science used to lengthen a person's lifespan) that I did two years ago. I was given only Kerala rice to eat twice a day and allowed milk from the cow that belonged to the Arya Vaidya Shala where I was living. I did not drink

the milk, but had milk substitutes. A paste of Ayurvedic herbs would arrive for me every evening. The treatment was a semi-fast for eighteen days. In the olden days, it was believed to regress ageing and promote vitality. I cannot even begin to tell you what I looked like and felt after I emerged from that treatment. In short, fasting really helps and if properly guided, works wonders!

As explained earlier, the liver is your master detox organ. Gut health, hormonal balance, weight loss and ageing are all connected to the liver. Out of all the organs, the liver is my favourite. It's like me—hardy and has resilience!

A detox doesn't mean your body gets rid of the toxins immediately; a real detox is done in phases. Why? This is because the liver also detoxes in two phases. In Phase 1, toxic wastes are converted into water-soluble compounds that can easily be eliminated into the bile to be carried to the digestive tract as waste or filtered through the kidneys. In Phase 2, products eliminated from Phase 1 are neutralized, wherein everything becomes water-soluble. Both Phase 1 and Phase 2 may need careful monitoring by a health practitioner. In Phase 1, protection of the liver cells is required by certain minerals like copper, manganese, zinc and vitamin C as free radicals (toxins) are flushed out. In Phase 2, nutrients like glutamine, choline, inositol and some antioxidants like vitamin E, coenzyme Q10 and vitamin C are helpful.

The detoxes in this book aim at supporting you with the right nutrients through the detox outlined in Phase 2, i.e., in the clean-out phase, building up to the master detox plan.

Just remember what we are aiming at is to get you back to a balanced pH.

Blood Condition and You

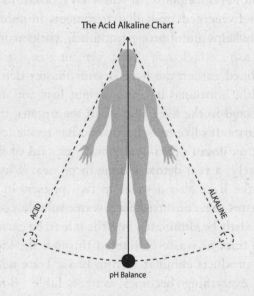

The Acid Alkaline Chart

ACID

ALKALINE

pH Balance

Remember yin and yang and these two polarities reflecting in everything? Well, even your body is acidic or alkaline. When the body fluid shows up as seven on your report (could be checked through your blood or urine), it shows the pH is neutral, which is what we would like it to be. At any given time, the blood condition can swing between acid and alkaline. Most of you will be acidic for sure; diet and environmental factors push you into this space. As much as

60 per cent of your diet should focus on alkaline foods, while the remaining 40 per cent on acid-forming foods. By this I don't mean junk foods and drink, but whole foods like brown rice, legumes, etc. Many dieticians and nutritionists would advise you to stay alkaline, but they forget that it's the right balance between acid and alkaline that you should achieve. After digesting both these type of foods, the body produces 'alkaline ash', which helps keep the internal environment healthy (basically promotes gut health). Your pH is off if:

(1) Your tongue is coated white in the morning when you wake up.
(2) You suffer from allergies, headaches, IBD, acid reflux or any other ailment.

Take this quiz to find out if you need a condensed juice/smoothie detox:

(1) Do you eat a lot of foods from a box, e.g., cookies, biscuits, etc.?

Yes   No

(2) Do you crave sugar often during the day?

Yes   No

(3) Do you crave tea/coffee often during the day?

Yes   No

(4) Have you been on medication/antibiotics for a long duration in your life?

Yes   No

(5) Women: Do you suffer from constant urinary tract infections (UTI)?

Yes   No

(6) Do you suffer from constant allergies?

Yes   No

(7) Do you weigh more than your average body weight?

Yes   No

(8) Do you have dark circles?

Yes   No

(9) Are you constantly tired?

Yes   No

(10) Are you generally constipated?

Yes   No

(11) Do you suffer from insomnia?

Yes   No

(12) Do you suffer from mental fuzziness?

Yes   No

Give yourself one point for every answer that is marked 'yes'. If you score under five, you are okay; anything over five and you could benefit from the juice detox outlined in Phase 1.

Good Gut Bite

Oil Pulling

It is a traditional Ayurvedic therapy that dates back to 3000 years, where oil (typically coconut or sesame [til]) is swished for twenty minutes in the mouth first thing in the morning, even before brushing your teeth. It is known to help with tooth issues, strengthens gums and jaw, improves acne, and also does away with microorganisms that cause bad breath. It helps with allergies, headaches and sinuses, reduces inflammation and boosts the immune system. Start with five minutes a day and then graduate to twenty minutes a day. It is an oral detoxification ritual that will help those on a detox. It's like using natural soap in your mouth every day.

ALKALINE FOODS CHART

MOSTLY ALKALINE	MODERTELY ALKALINE	SLIGHTLY ALKALINE	NEUTRAL
Celery	Beans (pulses, dahls)	Olives, eggplant	Ghee
Herbal teas	Beetroot, sprouts, avocados, bananas, broccoli	Brown rice, millet, buckwheat, black rice, coconut	Oils (except olive)
Watermelon, figs	Asparagus, cauliflower	Cucumber, honey (raw)	
Lemons	Green tea, radish, dates peas, peppers, pumpkin, turnips	Okra, onions, sesame, spices	
Mangoes	Kiwi, peaches, ginger, lettuce	Sprouted grains	
Papaya	Potatoes, corn, mushrooms, apple cider vinegar, umeboshi plum	Tangerines, tamari	
Grapes	Veggie juices	Radish	
Seaweed			

ACID-FORMING FOODS CHART

SLIGHTLY ACID-FORMING	MODERATELY ACID-FORMING	MOST ACID-FORMING
Eggs, kidney beans barley	Honey, bran, cheese	White bread, cakes, chocolate, yogurt (dairy)
Pumpkin and sesame seeds, butter	Dessicated coconut, goat's milk, pasta (whole grain)	Biscuits
Spinach	Grains (unrefined), mustard, prunes	Alcohol, soft drinks
	Popcorn, brown rice, tea, wheat	Artificial sweeteners, beef, pork, fish
		Sugar, dairy, molasses
		Table salt, Indian chai, walnuts
		Coffee, whole wheat
		Foods, antibiotics

PART THREE

INTRODUCTION

Phase 2 of the programme is where you will start the actual detox, so start by keeping all the foods specified in this phase away from the diet. These are: dairy, sugar, gluten, unhealthy fats, alcohol, antibiotics, eggs, sweeteners, diet sodas, aerated beverages, sauces, coffee, Indian tea, refined and processed foods; refined carbohydrates in the form of white rice, pasta, bread, cookies, biscuits, cakes; anything with preservatives, like fruit juices; and animal foods—fish, chicken and meat.

For those who are suffering from IBD-related ailments, please follow the cooked detox, and not the juice detox. For those who experience mild stomach issues, a half-cooked and half-juice approach may work. For some, a fully cooked detox, along with one green juice as a snack, will also work.

I recommend a three-day juice detox, followed by a cooked detox for the remaining duration of this phase, i.e., seven days. This makes it a total of ten days of detox for the clean-out phase of the programme. However, if you find it difficult to sustain a juice detox, which is literally a juice fast, please do the cooked detox right away and stick to it for ten days. For those of you who can sustain a seven-day juice detox (Jacqueline and I have done this together to support each other), go ahead, because it really works. But I must admit that it's not easy and takes a certain mindset to do it, but the results are amazing.

11

RAW DETOX JUICE DIET

Duration

The raw detox juice diet is for three or seven days. It is followed by the cooked detox to make up a total of ten days; so if you do a three-day juice detox, the cooked detox will be for seven days, and only for three days if you do a seven-day juice detox.

Juice Detox Chart with Timings for a Three or Seven-Day Detox

TIME	DAY 1	DAY 2	DAY 3
7 A.M.	GINGER TEA	GINGER TEA	GINGER TEA
8 A.M.	THE MORNING ENERGIZER	THE MORNING ENERGIZER	THE ANTI-INFLAMMATORY POWER JUICE
11 A.M.	THE MORNING ENERGIZER	THE MORNING ENERGIZER	THE MORNING ENERGIZER
2 P.M.	THE GLOW GIVER	THE GLOW GIVER	THE STRESS BUSTER
5 P.M.	THE ALKALIZER	THE ALKALIZER	THE ALKALIZER
8 P.M.	THE ANTI-INFLAMMATORY POWER JUICE	THE ANTI-INFLAMMATORY POWER JUICE	THE ALKALIZER
9 P.M.	NIGHTCAP	NIGHTCAP	NIGHTCAP

DAY 4	DAY 5	DAY 6	DAY 7
¬GER TEA	GINGER TEA	GINGER TEA	GINGER TEA
E MORNING ERGIZER	THE GLOW GIVER	THE STRESS BUSTER	THE MORNING ENERGIZER
E MORNING ERGIZER	THE GLOW GIVER	THE STRESS BUSTER	THE MORNING ENERGIZER
PER DETOX	SUPER DETOX	GOODNESS OF GREENS JUICE	THE STRESS BUSTER
E ANTI-INFLAMMATORY WER JUICE	THE MORNING ENERGIZER	BIO-PHOTONIC BOOST	THE VITAMIN C BOOST
E ANTI-INFLAMMATORY WER JUICE	THE THE MORNING ENERGIZER	BIO-PHOTONIC BOOST	BIO-PHOTONIC BOOST
GHTCAP	NIGHTCAP	NIGHTCAP	NIGHTCAP

Equipment

(1) A good mixer: Vitamix.
(2) A good cold-press juicer.
(3) Rubber spatula.
(4) Glass jars to work with and store in.
(5) Glass containers with holes or veggie bags with air holes for storage of vegetables.
(6) Glass bowls or jars to empty juices.

Tips

(1) Leave veggies (except greens) at room temperature before making a juice/smoothie.
(2) Don't store fruits and veggies together, as fruits give out ethylene as they ripen and this can spoil your veggies.
(3) Do not wash your herbs before storing, but only before juicing.
(4) Consume on an empty stomach.
(5) Wash berries or greens with vinegar and water (30:70).

Why Juice?

(1) It's a good way to have fruits and vegetables.
(2) Blending as opposed to juicing retains the fibre (or you can juice and add the fibre back). Having the fibre slows down carbohydrate digestion, thereby also controlling blood insulin levels.

(3) Highly concentrated source of vitamins, minerals and enzymes enter your bloodstream immediately (anything with 40 per cent and above greens has enough protein).

(4) Helps people with impaired digestion absorb nutrients better.

(5) Helps you rotate your veggies. Promotes weight loss.

(6) Increases vitamin C and potassium levels in the body.

(7) Lowers need for carbohydrates.

(8) Neutralizes body's pH levels; makes you more alkaline.

(9) Contains liquid sunshine, i.e., vitamin D and magnesium to calm you and your stomach muscles (when you take in leafy greens rich in chlorophyll).

Recipes

Method

Always juice the hard fruit or veggies, and blend the superfoods and avocado.

The Morning Energizer

- 2 apples (skinned and cut into wedges)
- ¼ pineapple chunk
- ¼ cucumber
- ¼ avocado
- 1 teaspoon spirulina
- ½ lime (peeled)
- 1 probiotic sachet (Econorm or Enterogermina from chemist)

The Glow Giver

- 2 apples (skinned and cut into wedges)
- ½ celery stick
- A large handful of leafy greens (mix rocket leaves and spinach)
- ½ cucumber
- 2 broccoli florets
- A small handful of sprouts
- 1 small chunk carrot
- ¼ inch beetroot
- ¼ inch zucchini
- A small piece of lemon rind
- ¼ inch ginger
- Ice

The Alkalizer

- ¼ small pineapple
- ½ inch cucumber
- ½ stick celery
- A small piece of lime
- 2 apples
- ¼ avocado
- A handful of greens
- Ice

The Anti-Inflammatory Power Juice

- 2 apples (skinned and cut into wedges)
- 2 carrots cut into chunks

- 1 inch lemon rind slice
- 2 inch ginger piece
- Ice

The Stress Buster

- ¼ pineapple
- 1 apple (skinned and cut into wedges)
- 200g yogurt (use soy yogurt if lactose intolerant or vegan)
- ½ teaspoon spirulina
- Ice

Super Detox

- 2 apples (skinned and cut into wedges)
- ½ cucumber
- 1 stick celery
- 1 tablespoon wheatgrass powder
- Ice

The Biophotonic Boost

- 2 apples (skinned and cut into wedges)
- ½ large pineapple
- ½ cup sprouts
- ½ cup parsley
- ½ cup kale
- 2–3 broccoli florets
- 1 teaspoon wheatgrass
- Ice

The Vitamin C Boost

- 2 apples (skinned and cut into wedges)
- ½ lemon
- Ice

Goodness of Greens Juice

- ½ cucumber
- 2 sticks celery
- A small handful of rocket
- 1 teaspoon spirulina
- 3 slices of orange
- Ice

Nightcap

- 3 apples
- 1 pinch ground cinnamon

Note: The method is different here. Juice these apples first. Boil it with a pinch of cinnamon powder in a saucepan. Have it as a nightcap.

Here Is a Peek into My Secret Superfood Cabinet

- Chia seeds (amazing fibre and omega-3—perfect for vegetarians); 1 tablespoon in any concoction. I use them in these ways:
  - In smoothies, as it is.

- o   Adding 1 tablespoon to seeds and a cinnamon stick to 1 litre of water. Soak it overnight and drink it in the first half of the day.
- o   The following day, use them in porridge, salads or in your flour dough when making chapattis.
- o   Add them to gravies by making a paste and blending it in.
- o   Coat cutlets with chia seeds and pan-fry them.
- o   Use chia seeds to substitute eggs. Add 1 tablespoon of chia to 3 tablespoons of water.
- o   If you bake, add it to pancakes, energy bars and cookies.

- Flax seeds or flax oil (great source of omega-3); 1 tablespoon in any concoction.
- A good protein powder (not whey or casein); ¼ tablespoon in any concoction.
- Maca powder or Peruvian ginseng (a root that belongs to the radish family, not native to India, but available online); ½ tablespoon in any concoction.
- Goji berries (native to India; rich in amino acids, B vitamins, and vitamins E and C); 1 tablespoon in any concoction.
- Raw cacao (raw chocolate superfood for weight loss and high energy. Rich in antioxidants such as manganese, iron, chromium, zinc, copper, vitamin C and tryptophan—a natural mood enhancer and crucial for seratonin, the feel-good hormone); 1 tablespoon in any concoction.
- Moringa powder (native to India, rich in amino acids [protein] and forty types of antioxidants and anti-inflammatory compounds); 1 heaped teaspoon in any concoction.

- Mixed seed blend (powerhouse in a small package): sunflower has all the essential fatty acids, amazing fibre, tryptophan, vitamin E and a whole lot more; pumpkin is rich in magnesium, zinc and omega-3. It is good for immune support, prostate health, aids the functioning of the heart and liver, and helps in the production of adenosine triphosphate (ATP).

Good Gut Bite

What Is ATP?

Adenosine triphosphate is responsible for intracellular exchange of energy transfer. Think of it as a currency used between cells to exchange energy. It is crucial for our survival on a cellular front. Your cells must absorb nutrients correctly in order to make ATP, and also use it as a radar to help them determine whether they should store or burn nutrients. In the case of cancers, for example, the ATP signal is not firing at optimum.

- Mixed nut blend: I generally blend almonds, walnuts and any one other nut.
- Hempseeds or oil (rich source of protein and enzymes, and an immunity booster); 1 tablespoon with any concoction (see Source List).
- A good probiotic supplement (specially for a detox) or you can add sauerkraut (see recipe); 1 heaped teaspoon.

- Basil or any herbs (for flavour).

Good Gut Bite

Amino Acids

There are some amino acids (building blocks of protein; 20 per cent of our body is made up of protein) that are absolutely critical for our well-being and vitality. Many factors prevent the utilization of amino acids in our bodies, such as a compromised digestive system, inflammation, bad diets, consuming foods with pesticides, smoking and drinking. It needs to be balanced right to speed up metabolism; we need to maintain the amino acid pool in the correct combination. There is a class of indispensable amino acids. These are: tryptophan, phenylalanine, methionine, valine, leucine, histidine and threonine. Some conditions also require arginine, cysteine, glutamine, tyrosine and proline. Sources of these are yogurt, paneer (eat only after rejuvenate phase), mushrooms, tempeh (fermented cultured soybean), cacao powder, whole bran, white oats (not rolled or steel cut), eggs, lentils, white beans, wheat germ, goat's cheese, green peas, amaranth (rajgeera) and quinoa.

Five Greens Juice Recipes You Must Try

Why Greens Juices?

(1) Chlorophyll, which is present in all green food, has anti-inflammatory and antimicrobial properties. It helps restore the body's pH. Chlorophyll's molecular structure is identical to haemoglobin. It is rich in vitamins A, C and E, and helps to bind and remove toxins.

(2) Chlorophyll contains magnesium, which the body needs to absorb vitamin D and calcium. Plus, it calms the digestive system and the muscles.

(3) Rotate your greens for greater benefits.

Bad Microbe Killer: Handful of rocket leaves + spinach, + ½ tomato + fistful of coriander + 1–2 carrots

- Releases stored toxins from processed foods.
- Helps in flushing out the toxins built up due to undigested foods.
- Rich in vitamin A; also includes vitamins K, C and B vitamins.

Divine Detox Mojito: 1 cucumber+ 1 pear + fistful of mint + 1 lime

- Contains minerals that are good for skin and hair.
- Pear flavonoids and phytochemicals help improve and stabilize digestion.

- Lime optimizes your pH.
- Mint boosts chlorophyll.

The Lung Cleanser: 1 lotus root + 1-inch ginger piece + 1 apple + handful of kale + 1 lemon

- Cleans lungs (mucous, phlegm).
- Kale contains forty-five different antioxidant flavonoids and is anti-inflammatory.
- Apple, lemon and ginger balance pH.

The Alkalizer: Handful of kale + 1 cucumber + 2 celery + 1 apple + 1 lemon + ½-inch piece of ginger

- Cucumber provides hydration.
- Celery provides loads of free-radical fighters.
- Lemon fights fat.
- Ginger aids digestion.
- Kale adds proteins, keeping you satiated.

De-Bloat Juice: 2 celery + 1 cucumber + 1 teaspoon of wheatgrass + 1 orange

- Wheatgrass increases oxygen, making you feel alive and vibrant.
- Oranges add vitamin C.

Use the above greens juices any time during your detox phase—it's great for the liver, as the liver loves greens. You can interchange a juice from the juice detox chart with any one of the juices mentioned above for a change. Adding an extra greens juice always boosts the detox.

Follow these tips to make the juice detox easier:

(1) If you feel hungry, eat fruits between meals or raw vegetables like carrots, celery and cucumber.

(2) Drink green or herbal teas.

(3) Hydrate regularly, especially with the 'diet detox boost water' (recipe provided later in this book), rejuvelac drink (recipe provided later), water, herbal teas or one vegetable juice.

(4) Practise deep breathing.

(5) Meditate.

(6) Do some light exercise—yoga or stretching.

(7) Take time out for body scrubbing.

(8) Include a magnesium supplement (calms the bowels).

(9) Include a probiotic supplement daily (see Source List).

(10) Sit in the sun for twenty minutes to increase vitamin D; if this is difficult, take a vitamin D3 supplement.

12

REGENERATION DETOX DIET

Duration

For three days if you do a juice detox for seven days, for seven days if you do a juice detox for three days, and for ten days if you have IBD, i.e., no juice detox for you.

The goal of this phase is to provide you with energy and nutrients to rebuild your body. At the end of this phase, your soldiers, i.e., the white blood cells would have been renewed. You will feel detoxified and your digestive system will be alive with good gut microbes.

Day 1

Breakfast

- Lemon ginger tea
- Soup with leafy greens (add 1 teaspoon miso paste after cooking)

Lunch

- Pressed salad (mix of vegetables)
- Sauerkraut

Snack

- One portion of fruit (stewed)

Dinner

- Soup with miso (add 2 tablespoons of cooked millet and blend it in the soup)
- Blanched vegetables
- Pickles

Day 2

Breakfast

- Lemon ginger tea
- Soup (add 1 teaspoon miso after cooking) with leafy greens

Lunch

- Pressed salad
- Green salad (with only lime dressing)

Snack

- One portion of fruit (stewed)

Dinner

- Soup with miso
- Steamed vegetables
- Sauerkraut

Day 3

Breakfast

- Lemon ginger tea
- Miso (add 1 teaspoon miso after cooking) soup with leafy greens

Lunch

- Quick-pickled radishes
- Mixed vegetable soup with miso

Snack

- One portion of fruit (stewed)

Dinner

- Soup with miso
- Boiled vegetable salad with lime and sesame seeds
- Sauerkraut

Day 4

Breakfast

- Lemon ginger tea
- Brown rice porridge (made with kombu)

Lunch

- Millet couscous
- Pressed salad
- Nishime-style vegetables

Snack

- One portion of fruit

Dinner

- Soup with miso
- Brown rice mixed with any bean (white, red or black kidney)
- Boiled vegetable salad with lime and sesame seeds
- Pressed salad (saved from afternoon)

Day 5

Breakfast

- Lemon ginger tea
- Vegetable soup with cooked millet (3 tablespoons) and miso paste

Lunch

- Blanched and steamed vegetable salad
- Sauerkraut (2 tablespoons)
- Brown rice
- Yellow mung dahl or sprouts sautéed in coconut oil with mustard seeds and curry leaves

Snack

- One portion of fruit (stewed)

Dinner

- Soup with miso
- Boiled vegetable salad with lime and sesame seeds
- Sauerkraut

Day 6

Breakfast

- Lemon ginger tea
- Brown rice porridge

Lunch

- Millet, poha-style or couscous-style
- Steamed vegetables with lemon tahini sauce
- Mixed vegetable soup with miso
- Pickles

Snack

- One portion of fruit (stewed)

Dinner

- Soup with miso
- Nishime
- Boiled vegetable salad
- Sauerkraut

Day 7

Breakfast

- Lemon ginger tea
- Millet poha or porridge

Lunch

- Steamed vegetable salad
- Quick-pickled radishes
- Brown rice mixed with sprouts

Snack

- One portion of fruit (stewed)

Dinner

- Soup with miso
- Boiled vegetable salad with lime and sesame seeds
- Sauerkraut

The Detox Diet Boost Water

Ingredients

- 1-inch piece of ginger, grated
- Juice of one lime
- Few slivers of fresh haldi
- 4 cups of water

Method

Boil water and add ginger and haldi. Simmer for 4–5 minutes. Cool down and add lime juice. Cool and store to be sipped throughout the day. The water will increase metabolism and support digestion.

What You Can Expect from This Detox

This time you will observe the following: Strength in the gut, greater mental clarity, release of old emotions, clearing up off stagnant patterns, shift in energy levels, happier state of mind, aches and pains disappearing, and a shift in your weight.

What you should be prepared for during the detox: Minor cold, cough, loose stomach, headaches, body odour and uncomfortable thoughts. It's always good to be in a quiet phase on a detox.

Contraindications: Some of you may find it difficult to take in the new foods, especially those used to eating animal protein. If you feel tired and look pale, increase the quotient of leafy greens during this phase and add some fish to widen the detox plan (usually steamed or boiled). Avoid frying or baking fish.

Follow these tips to enhance the effects of the regeneration detox:

(1) Drink fluids, especially the diet detox boost water and rejuvelac drink (see recipe below), along with water, herbal teas and one vegetable juice.
(2) Practise deep breathing.
(3) Meditate.
(4) Do some light exercise—yoga or stretching.
(5) Indulge in body scrubbing.
(6) To maintain healthy bowel movements, add ½ heaped tablespoon (heaped) of Vaiswanara Choornam (see Source List) in water and drink it before bedtime.
(7) Add inulin in powder form (see Source List).
(8) Have a vitamin C supplement (3–8g [not all at once]). It's a laxative.
(9) Include a magnesium supplement (calms the bowels).
(10) Include a probiotic supplement daily (see Source List).
(11) Sit in the sun for twenty minutes to increase vitamin D. If this is difficult, take a vitamin D3 supplement.

What Benefits the Liver during a Cleanse?

(1) Stretching: The liver controls the tendons. According to TCM, the liver stores blood during periods of rest and then releases it. It is connected to the tendons in times of activity, maintaining tendon health and flexibility. So incorporate a morning stretch into your routine. Try yoga or tai chi.

(2) Eye exercises: Although all organs are related to the health of the eyes, the liver is linked to proper eye function. Remember to take breaks when looking at a computer monitor for extended periods of time and do eye exercises. Practise staring at an object for a minute and above or try candle gazing.

(3) Eating greens: Green is the colour of the liver and of springtime (also associated with the liver). Eating young plants—fresh, leafy greens, sprouts and immature cereal grasses—can improve the liver's overall function and aid in the movement of qi.

(4) Eating sour food: Sour food and drinks are thought to stimulate the liver's qi. Put lemon slices in your drinking water, and use vinegar and olive oil for your salad dressing. Garnish your sandwich with a slice of dill pickle.

(5) Doing more outdoor activities: Outside air helps the qi flow of the liver. If you have been feeling irritable, find an outdoor activity to smooth out that liver qi stagnation. Try hiking, trekking, running or take up golf.

(6) Drinking milk-thistle tea: Milk thistle helps protect the liver cells from incoming toxins and encourages the liver

to cleanse itself of damaging substances, such as alcohol, medications, pesticides, environmental toxins and even heavy metals such as mercury.

(7) Getting acupuncture treatments: Acupuncture and oriental medicine can help improve the overall health of your liver as well as treat stress, anger and frustration, which are often associated with liver qi disharmony.

Frequently Asked Questions (FAQs)

Here are some FAQs that have emerged from my detox workshops about this phase:

Q. If I have a headache, what do I do?
A. Have a green tea.

Q. Is regular coffee or tea allowed on a cleanse?
A. No.

Q. Is fresh lime water okay to drink?
A. Yes. No honey, sugar or sea/rock salt is allowed.

Q. Can I have a grain in one meal?
A. Yes, if you feel you are getting a headache.

Q. Is it okay to have any fruit?

A. Yes, except bananas. Also, use fruit as a snack between meals.

Q. Can I have blanched mushrooms?

A. Yes.

Q. Is it okay to have roasted *makhana* with sea salt?

A. No.

Q. What is the best snack I can eat?

A. Sweet potato with lime (boiled and cubed or mashed).

Q. How should I make my food interesting?

A. Use the sauces in the Recipe section on veggies.

13

THE MASTER DETOX DIET

Duration

The master detox diet is for four weeks; twelve if problems are severe. It is not just a diet, but an approach to eating. For many, this could become a way of life, while others might want to try it out for 4–12 weeks (depending on the nature of your issues), and then start introducing the foods that you were used to.

This is the diet for the Rejuvenate phase of your detox journey. To reiterate, remember that the focus here is to eat the MACs. These are: whole grains, vegetables, fruits, legumes, nuts, seeds, healthy fats, oily fish, good fermented products, prebiotics, sprouts, bone soups (of course the fish and bone soups are for non-vegetarians). Remember that foods from the top-it-up phase need to be added in the fourth week of this diet. I will try to incorporate it all in your diet plan, and wherever you need supplements, I will mention it. While I outline a one-week plan, you need to replicate or add other foods, based on the basic food groups like whole grain, legumes or fish, some chicken, vegetables, good fermented products, fruits, nuts and seeds, bone broths, soups and herbal teas. You will still stay off the foods mentioned in the clean-out phase of the diet.

The main goal of this phase is to improve the diversity of your gut bacteria and increase the amount of SCFAs produced through bacterial fermentation. I have to thank the Sonnenbergs again for bringing the MACs to the forefront, as these will form the core of this phase. The key here is to maintain the diet over time if you really want to improve your health, and of course, change the gut population of diverse strains of bacteria.

Day 1

Breakfast

- Lemon ginger tea
- **Indian breakfast:** Good-gut brown-rice poha with carrots and sweet potatoes with ½ cup finely chopped sauerkraut

or

Western breakfast: Millet, porridge-style, with almond milk (same recipe as brown-rice porridge), stewed apples with walnuts and 1 tablespoon of mounaka raisins or bacteria-boosting banana strawberry smoothie

Lunch

- Radish, red grape and rocket leaf/arugula salad with two tablespoons cooked millet
- 2 tablespoons pressed salad (mix of vegetables)—any recipe from fermented foods in the Recipe section can be used. You need to have up to 2 tablespoons of a fermented food in every meal.
- Almost chilled kefir berry soup (see cold soup recipes)

Snack

- Fruit (the following are prebiotic: bananas, apples, blueberries, pears, melons, peaches and strawberries), rejuvelac (flavour it with lime juice or some homemade cold-brewed tea; it becomes easier to drink with flavouring) or kanji (½ glass)

Dinner

- Soup with miso paste (1 teaspoon miso paste is added per serving, once the soup has been cooked. Please add a bone soup (see recipes) daily at dinner if you are a non-vegetarian and feel your condition is severe and you suffer from leaky gut syndrome)
- **Indian dinner:** 2 chapattis (amaranth [rajgeera] and jowar mixed) with vegetables: red, yellow and green bell peppers, and tofu (Indian)

or

Western dinner: Gluten-free pasta with my mushroom marinara sauce and vegetables: red, yellow, green bell peppers, and tofu/fish

- Pickles or any recipe from fermented foods in the Recipe section of the book

Fibre: Approximately 35g

Day 2

Breakfast

- Lemon ginger tea

- **Indian breakfast:** Millet poha with steamed cabbage and grated carrots with ½ cup of finely chopped sauerkraut

or

Western breakfast: Brown-rice porridge or chlorophyll-rich green smoothie

Lunch

- Antioxidant-rich chickpea peppery salad and 2 tablespoons of cooked millet
- 2 tablespoons of papaya khimchi

Snack

- Fruit with rejuvelac, chilled berry soup or kanji (½ glass)

Dinner

- Soup with miso
- **Indian dinner:** Millet made like cumin (jeera) rice and vegetables: doodhi (bottle gourd) gravy and yellow mung dahl

or

Western dinner: MAC-rich mint couscous with vegetables, steamed fish, steamed/boiled sweet potato and broccoli with lemon tahini sauce

Fibre: Approximately 39g

Day 3

Breakfast

- Lemon ginger tea
- Steel-cut oats with vegetables (savoury) or with almond milk (sweet), and stewed apples with ½ cup of finely chopped sauerkraut

or

Golden-glow papaya and banana smoothie

Lunch

- **Indian lunch:** Millet (khichdi-style gravy with red pumpkin and *kasoori* methi) with organism-fuelled Odessa beet salad and steamed sprouts

or

Western lunch: Stir-fried tofu and black bean. Add 2 tablespoons of cooked millet and steamed vegetables with green heaven dip (blended with white miso)

- Beetroot pickle (4 pieces)

Snack

- Fruit + rejuvelac or kanji (½ glass)

Dinner

- Soup with miso
- **Indian lunch:** Brown-rice croquettes with vegetables: prebiotic-powered sweet potato and broccoli, and yellow mung dahl

or

Western lunch: Brown-rice cutlets with steamed fish, red pepper and nut salsa, and baked eggplant

Fibre: Approximately 33g

Day 4

Breakfast

- Lemon ginger tea
- Jowar khakra (2 home-made Indian flatbread) with chopped avocado and home-made salsa with ½ cup of finely chopped sauerkraut or antioxidant pomegranate stress buster

Lunch

- **Indian lunch:** Brown jeera rice with turai and mixed dahl (add miso paste to dahl)

or

Western lunch: Tabbouleh-style millet, made with foxtail or kodo millet or quinoa and red pumpkin in a gravy

- 2 tablespoons of turmeric pickle

Snack

- Fruit + rejuvelac or kanji (½ glass)

Dinner

- Soup with miso
- **Indian dinner:** Millet (curry leaves and mustard seeds) with spinach and sprouts in gravy

or

Western dinner: Vegetable pasta (tomato-base pasta sauce) with MAC-rich mint couscous and vegetables, and fats-galore fish burgers

Fibre: Approximately 35g

Day 5

Breakfast

- Lemon ginger tea
- Brown-rice porridge (sweet or savoury with vegetables) or centering brown-rice idlis with coconut chutney and sweet potato vegetable masala with ½ cup of finely chopped sauerkraut

or

Good-bug mixed fruit and berry smoothie

Lunch

- **Indian lunch:** Amaranth (rajgeera) and 2 sorghum (jowar) *paranthas* with soy yogurt (raita-style, flavoured with cumin powder and sea/rock salt), and pickles

or

Western lunch: Flavourful soba noodles (with miso) and vegetables
- 2 tablespoons of pressed salad

Snack

- Fruit + kanji or rejuvelac (½ glass)

or

Hummus (mixed with white miso) with veggie sticks of carrot and cucumber

Dinner

- Probiotic pumpkin soup with 2 tablespoons of cooked grain (millet)
- Vegetables
- Asian salmon with succulent sweet potato pickle

Fibre: Approximately 36g

Day 6

Breakfast

- Lemon ginger tea
- Green heaven smoothie

Lunch

- **Indian lunch:** Corn (*makai*) rotis with spinach (*palak* or saag or Malabar spinach), white *urad* dahl (dry) and chilled cucumber yogurt soup

or

Western lunch: Corn tortillas with microbiota-rich marinated bell peppers and refried beans, and tofu sour cream

- 2 tablespoons of ginger pickle

Snack

- Fruit and rejuvelac or kanji (½ glass)

Dinner

- Soup with miso
- **Indian dinner:** Brown rice with yellow mung dahl and *parwal* stuffed with sweet potato

or

Western dinner: Quiet-stomach quinoa pilaf with nishime vegetables and steamed fish, and red pepper nut salsa

Fibre: Approximately 39g

Day 7

Breakfast

- Lemon ginger tea
- Steel-cut oats with vegetables (savoury) or with almond milk (sweet) and stewed apples with ½ cup of finely chopped sauerkraut

or

Chlorophyll-rich green smoothie

Lunch

- **Indian lunch:** Amaranth (rajgeera) and sorghum (jowar) rotis, mixed vegetable cutlet and tomato salsa or green coriander chutney (add miso)

or

Western lunch: Crispy rotis (made flat like pizza dough) topped with chopped pickles or sauerkraut, tomato salsa, guacamole and sprouts (for vegetarians)/sardines for non-vegetarians with chilled marinated bell peppers and tofu sour cream

Snack

- Fruit + rejuvelac or kanji (½ glass)

Dinner

- Fish and noodle soup

or

Belly-up round vegetable soup with miso

- Barley and mushroom risotto and L-glutamine-rich two-tone coleslaw (mix 2 tablespoons sauerkraut in coleslaw)

Fibre: Approximately 39g

To continue the detox for another three weeks, you have to maintain the same format, including whole grains like brown rice, millets and millet flours, which are gluten-free in pastas. For an Indian meal, include legumes: whole beans and dahls; vegetables: all; focus on the prebiotic ones and add a lot of leafy greens; and 1–2 fermented foods daily. I reiterate, stay clear of the foods mentioned in the clean-out phase of this plan.

Use the following tips to adapt to the diet:

(1) For those who have sugar cravings, add a sweet vegetable drink (see recipe) in the late afternoons.

(2) For those who have a serious stomach issue, take *ume sho kudzu* at bedtime for ten days, then take a break for three days and repeat again for ten days. Continue in this manner for one month.

(3) For those who suffer from mild stomach issues or even anxiety, have an apple kudzu drink at bedtime.

(4) Hydrate with the 'diet detox boost water', rejuvelac drink (see recipe), water and herbal teas.

(5) If you feel hungry, add a green juice as a snack.

(6) Drink the concoction of brewer's yeast added to water daily (1–2 tablespoons in one glass of water).

(7) Add inulin in powder form (see Source List).

(8) L-glutamine helps with leaky gut and supports the immune system.

(9) You can add 1–2 teaspoons of manuka honey to your diet, as it destroys the *Helicobacter pylori* bacteria.

(10) Add a CoQ10 supplement.

(11) Add B complex.

(12) Add ashwagandha (see Source List).

(13) Add shilajit (see Source List).

(14) For healthy bowel movements, use Vaiswanara Choornam (see Source List: order from Arya Vaidya Pharmacy). Have ½ heaped tablespoon with water before bedtime.

(15) Have 3–8g of vitamin C supplement (not all at once).

(16) Include a magnesium supplement.

(17) Include a probiotic supplement daily (see Source List).

(18) Try and do as much as you can from the Oxygenate chapter of this book.

Discharge That You Can Expect During the Detox Process

(1) **Headaches:** These are normal for people who stop having coffee or Indian tea, which have caffeine. The way to combat this is to substitute it with green tea.

(2) **Increased Cravings:** This is normal as the 'monkey mind' plays tricks on you and the body goes into a withdrawal mode. Stay with it; don't cave in.

(3) **Tiredness:** This will happen as the blood sugar levels adjust to a new diet. This should disappear in 2–3 days.

(4) **Cold:** Also a sign that the body is getting ready to rid itself of excess mucous.

(5) **Body odour:** The food discharge happens through pores also (that's why a body scrub is recommended), so your pH balance may change and reflect in the smell of your sweat. This is normal, so stay with it; once the detox starts having an effect, this will come back to normal.

(6) **Strong emotions:** This is also normal, as you are not only cleansing the physical body but also the mind. The energies get lighter as opposed to you

being heavy and dense. This will or may lead to a discharge of negative emotions.

(7) **Fever:** The body may throw up old foods (in urine, sweat and stools) and you may get a fever to combat the detoxification process.

The Detox Pantry

(1) **Whole grain:** Brown rice, red rice and all millets, specifically—foxtail (cheena), kodo, barnyard, sorghum (jowar), finger millet (ragi/nachni), whole barley and buckwheat (*kuttu*).

(2) **Pseudo-grains:** Amaranth (rajgeera) and quinoa.

(3) **Legumes:** Whole beans like chickpeas, red or black kidney beans, white beans (lobhia), green mung and all split lentils like pigeon pea (*tuvar*), gram (*chana*) and yellow mung.

(4) **Fish:** All oily fish and white meat fish.

(5) **Vegetables:** Beetroot, Brussel sprouts, broccoli, bok choy, cabbage, cauliflower, carrots, celery, cholai (amaranth leaves), cucumber, eggplant (*baigan*), fenugreek (methi), garlic, ginger, bottle gourd (doodhi), kale, lettuce, lotus root (bhen), mushrooms, okra (bhindi), parwal, peppers (red, green and yellow), rocket leaves (arugula), snake gourd (turai), spinach (palak), squash, tomatoes and turnips (shalgham).

(6) **Fruits:** All seasonal fruits.

(7) **Nuts:** Almonds, walnuts, pine nuts and Brazil nuts. Minimize consumption of cashews and peanuts.

(8) **Oils:** All cold-pressed oils: olive, sesame, mustard, coconut oil, flaxseed oil and also ghee.

(9) **Fermented foods:** Quick pickles, sauerkrauts, kombucha, kanji and rejuvelac (see Recipe section for more).

(10) **Seeds:** Chia, flax, sesame (especially *gomashio*— see recipe), sunflower, pumpkin and melon

What Do You Do Once You Are Done with the Rejuvenate Phase of the Diet?

You can follow the dietary recommendations of the phase and continue it, or choose to be 90 per cent compliant. I am sure that by the end of this phase, the gut lining would have been repaired and your tolerance to the foods you were used to eating before would have gone up. One way of measuring how you feel is to have the food and let your gut respond. You will know immediately.

Manju came to me with ulcerative colitis. She was based in London, so we worked together long-distance to solve her issues. I put her on the programme, and she followed it strictly for eight months. After six months, she went to her doctors for a check-up and found that the first two linings of her intestine had completely healed. The doctors were shocked. After eight months, she asked me if she could drink a glass of wine (she loved having her one glass every day) and a bit of aged cheese. I was taught by my macrobiotic teacher John Kozinski to follow a 'wide' macrobiotic approach and not be 'narrow'. So I told her to watch out for her symptoms, and go ahead if she wanted to.

She is fine to this date, which is six years after her initial diagnosis. This only goes to show that the intestinal lining has the capacity to heal, and that once it does, you can live normally, indulging from time to time.

I still do not recommend dairy. However, if you can get your hands on goat's milk, go ahead. So here is the list of recommended foods for your daily diet and lifestyle:

(1)   Eggs: preferably free-range eggs (you get them at the local speciality food stores [see Source List])

(2)   Gluten-free grains: brown rice, red rice, sorghum (jowar), foxtail (cheena), kodo, barnyard, finger millet (ragi/nachni), whole barley, buckwheat (kuttu) and oats (steel-cut or whole)

(3)   Pseudo-grains: amaranth (rajgeera) and quinoa (these two come from a family of grasses, therefore referred to as pseudo-grains and not whole grains)

(4)   Meats in moderation

(5)   Chicken in moderation

(6)   Legumes

(7)   Vegetables

(8)   Good-quality fermented foods

(9)   Beverages: tea (occasional), coffee (occasional); try sticking to herbal tea

(10) Nuts

(11) Seeds

(12) Dry fruits (occasional)

(13) Stevia

(14) Manuka honey

(15) Dark chocolate

Minimize the use of alcohol and avoid processed and refined foods, colas, aerated drinks, coffee, tea, sugar, dairy/dairy products, sweeteners, white processed flour (maida), foods out of a box (biscuits/cookies), commercial bread, preservatives, commercial honey, fruit juices (take it only occasionally), excessive use of dried fruits, foods with high corn fructose syrup, hydrogenated fats and trans fats, and food with preservatives, added colours and food enhancers (this includes MSG in foods).

PART FOUR

14

RECIPES

Breakfast

Good-Gut Brown-Rice Poha with Carrots or Sweet Potatoes (Serves 6)

Ingredients

4 cups brown or red rice poha
1 medium sweet potato, grated medium fine
6 tablespoons cold-pressed oil/ghee
1 teaspoon cumin seeds
½ teaspoon mustard seeds
1 pinch of asafoetida
10 curry leaves, fresh or dried
1 small handful of cilantro leaves, chopped
1 small green chilli, chopped
1 small onion, chopped fine
1 teaspoon turmeric

1 handful of peanuts, roasted
½ teaspoon rock or sea salt

Method

1. Soak the poha, if brown; wash and keep wet, if red.
2. Heat oil/ghee in a frying pan. When hot, add cumin seeds, mustard seeds, curry leaves and asafoetida. Let the seeds pop.
3. Add cilantro, chilli and onion.
4. Cook over medium heat until the onions are translucent, stirring occasionally to prevent it from sticking.
5. Add grated potato. Stir well, cover and cook for five minutes. Stir well again and cook for another five minutes.
6. Add salt, turmeric and poha at the end of five minutes. Mix well. Cover and turn off heat, and let it sit for a few minutes.
7. Garnish with roasted peanuts.

Yummiest Brown-Rice Porridge (Serves 1)

The sweetness of the porridge comes from the apples.

Ingredients

½ cup cooked brown rice (leftover rice works great for this)

¼ cup water or almond milk (don't use nuts if you are using almond milk)
1 tablespoon mounaka raisins
½ apple cut into four and sliced thin and long
1 tablespoon walnuts, roasted and chopped
1 tablespoon almonds, roasted and chopped
A dash of cinnamon

Method

1. Blend cooked (leftover) brown rice with water or almond milk. Don't blend it fine; keep it grainy.
2. In the meantime, keep apples to stew with a little water and a dash of cinnamon.
3. Put brown rice in a porridge bowl, layer with apples, add mounaka raisins and top it with nuts.

Note: You can substitute brown rice with millet (foxtail or cheena).

Centering Brown-Rice Idlis (Makes 16 Idlis)

Ingredients

¾ cup brown rice, soaked in the morning
¼ cup white urad dahl, soaked in the morning
1 tablespoon white miso paste

Note: The ingredients require soaking for an entire day. Then grind the grains and lentil into a smooth batter and leave it for fermenting overnight.

Method

1. Grind both rice and urad dahl in the evening and mix together.
2. Must be ground extra fine, should not be grainy.
3. Add 1 tablespoon white miso to this batter.
4. Ferment overnight.
5. The batter is ready to use the next morning.

Other Breakfast Options

(1) Dosas
(2) Pancakes made with idli batter (can be had with honey)
(3) Polenta (corn grits) made like upma
(4) Soup with whole grain and veggies thrown into it or grain-blended soup (especially in winter); don't forget to add 1 teaspoon miso paste in the end
(5) Home-made bread once a week with a spread of your choice or chopped avocados and tomatoes (this could also be done on home-made khakras)

Almond Milk (Makes 4–5 Cups)

Ingredients

1 cup almonds, soaked
4 cups water

Method

1. Place water and almonds in a blender.

2. Sieve it through a muslin or cheesecloth to remove the milk.
3. Save almond residue and use in rotis (Indian flatbread), to top cereal, vegetables or rice, or in smoothies.

Note: Alternatively, to make the milk thick, you can keep almonds and water in a jar in the fridge for two days and then blend it together.

Smoothies/Juices

Gratifying Green Juice (Serves 2)

Get your daily dose of greens with this juice. Makes for a great filler between meals.

Ingredients

½ bottle gourd (*lauki*)
2 carrots
½ cup water or vegetable stock
2-inch piece ginger
1 tablespoon spirulina powder
2 teaspoons lemon juice
1 teaspoon wheatgrass powder
¼ cup sauerkraut

Method

1. Put the vegetables and water/stock in a blender, and blend until smooth.

2. Add all other ingredients and blend again until smooth.
3. Pour into glasses and enjoy!

Bacteria-Boosting Banana Strawberry Smoothie (Serves 2)

Ingredients

⅔ cup yogurt or soy yogurt
1½ cup coconut milk
1 teaspoon chia seeds
2 bananas
2 cups strawberries

Method

Blend all the above ingredients till creamy.

Chlorophyll-Rich Green Smoothie (Serves 1)

Ingredients

1 ripe banana, frozen
2 handfuls leafy greens
1¼ cups soy or almond milk
¼ avocado
1 tablespoon chia seeds
3 dates
¼ cup sauerkraut
Handful of ice

Method

1. Blend all the ingredients until smooth and creamy.
2. Add the milk (almond or soy) to thin it down.

Golden-Glow Papaya and Banana Smoothie (Serves 2)

Ingredients

1 banana, cut into sizeable chunks
½ papaya, cut into sizeable chunks
½ cup soy yogurt
1 teaspoon spirulina (optional)

Method

Blend all the above ingredients till creamy.

Antioxidant Pomegranate Stress Buster (Serves 2)

Ingredients

2 pomegranates
2 oranges (optional)
Some ice
1 teaspoon chia seeds
¼ cup sauerkraut

Method

Put pomegranate seeds in a juicer. If you are using oranges, use a citrus juicer to extract the juice, blend together all the ingredients and pour over ice.

Good-Bug Mixed-Fruit and Berry Smoothie (Serves 2)

Ingredients

½ cup berries (any)
2 tablespoons pomegranate seeds
1 tablespoon sunflower or pumpkin seeds (unsalted)
1 teaspoon flaxseeds
1 apple
½ papaya or 1 mango (if in season)
½ teaspoon wheatgrass powder
½ cup coconut milk
¼ cup sauerkraut

Method

Blend all the ingredients in a blender and pour over ice.

Soups

Basic Vegetable Stock for Soups and Curries (Servings: 12 cups)

Ingredients

4 celery stalks, cut small
2 onions, diced
4 cloves of garlic, peeled and cut small
3–4 carrots cubed
2 cups mushrooms, chopped

A handful of parsley
4 bay leaves (tej patta)
Sea salt
16 cups of water

Method

1. Add onions, garlic and sea salt in a large vessel. Add 1 cup of water initially and let it simmer for about ten minutes after the first boil.
2. Add the remaining vegetables, water and bring to a boil.
3. Reduce heat and cook on a low fire for about one hour, so that the liquid boils down to about 12 cups.
4. Run water through a sieve, press down vegetables to squeeze out water and either discard the vegetables or use it in a soup.

Note: I use this stock for all my soups, some vegetable curries and some cold vegetable drinks as well.

Sweet Miso Soup (Servings: 12)

Ingredients

8 cups water or vegetable stock
1 small squash or red pumpkin (bhopla), cubed
1 medium onion, cut into thin rounds
1 small white radish cut into thin rounds

6 tablespoons white or barley miso
1 green onion stalk sliced fine for garnish
Parsley for garnishing

Method

1. Bring 8 cups of water/stock to a boil.
2. Add onion to pot. Simmer uncovered for five minutes. Add the radish and simmer for another five minutes.
3. Add the squash and simmer till it is tender (about five more minutes). Remove from heat.
4. Place a small amount of the hot soup in a small bowl, add the miso, whisk till smooth and return to pot. Stir and garnish with green onions (this is the standard way to mix in the miso).
5. Garnish with parsley.

Note: Do not boil soup again after adding miso as the beneficial microorganisms that will aid digestion get destroyed.

Bacteria-Rich Broccoli Soup (Servings: 2–4)

Ingredients

5 cups of water or vegetable stock (enhances nutrient value)
1½ cups chopped broccoli
1 small onion, cut really fine

½ sweet potato, cubed; adds great texture to the soup and makes for sweetness

1½ cups cooked brown rice

2 tablespoons miso—always use a lighter miso for children as darker versions have stronger taste

Use some steamed broccoli florets, chopped into small pieces, for garnishing

Method

1. Add broccoli, sweet potato and onion to the water/vegetable stock and bring to a boil (or pressure-cook).
2. Cover and simmer for ten minutes.
3. After vegetables are tender, cool the liquid and use a hand blender to mix in the brown rice. This is an especially good technique to camouflage the brown rice for children and get it into their diet.
4. Mix 1–2 tablespoons of miso in the soup (by mixing separately in a cup and adding to soup).
5. Garnish with broccoli.

Note: You can use celery or lettuce instead of broccoli.

Fresh Corn Chowder Soup (Servings: 6 cups)

Ingredients

1 onion, diced
2 medium celery stalks, chopped fine
6 corns, shelled

1 large sweet potato, cubed
4 cups vegetable stock or water
3 tablespoons light miso
1½ teaspoon salt
½ teaspoon black pepper
Parsley/coriander for garnishing

Method

1. Place the onion, celery stalks, corn and sweet potatoes in stock or water.
2. Bring to a boil, reduce heat and simmer (covered) till potatoes are tender. It should take 10–15 minutes.
3. Add 1½ teaspoons salt and ½ teaspoon black pepper. Simmer for about five more minutes. Blend in a mixer after cooling and return to heat for one more boil.
4. Add 3 tablespoons of light miso.
5. Garnish with parsley or coriander.

Belly-Up Round Vegetable Soup (Servings: 4)

It has tremendous calming energy and makes for a satisfied feeling in your belly!

Ingredients

½ cup yam (*suran*), cubed
2 turnips (*shalgam*), cubed

3–4 colocasia (*arbi*), cut small
2 carrots, diced
1 white radish, cut small
1 onion, sliced long and thin
3–4 cinnamon sticks
3–4 cloves
1 tablespoon curry powder
4 teaspoons dark or light miso
1 tablespoon olive oil
3 cups of water or vegetable stock
3 tablespoons miso paste
Parsley for garnishing

Method

1. Add the oil to a soup pot. Before it heats up, add onions, cinnamon and cloves. Sauté till onions are a little soft.
2. Add vegetables in the following order: turnips, yam, colocasia, white radish and carrots.
3. Sauté for ten minutes and then add the curry powder.
4. Add water/stock. After the first boil, simmer on low heat for twenty minutes.
5. Once the vegetables are tender, blend them with a hand blender.
6. Take out a little soup in a cup, add the miso, mix well and put it in the soup pot. Give it a good stir.
7. Garnish with parsley.

Fibre-Friendly Hearty Brown Rice Soup (Servings: 6)

Brown rice provides sustained sugars and has a complete nutritional profile, with all the necessary minerals and vitamins one would need on a detox. Besides, it's a great source of fibre to clean up the intestines—necessary while on a detox.

Ingredients

1 cup chopped onions
1 tablespoon olive oil
1 cup cooked brown rice
A pinch each of thyme, marjoram and sea salt
8 cups of vegetable stock or boiling water
1 tablespoon soy sauce
1 cup cooked chickpeas
3 tablespoons miso paste

Method

1. In a skillet, sauté the onions in olive oil over medium heat until translucent.
2. In a large saucepan, combine onions with all the rest of the ingredients and bring to a boil. Reduce heat and simmer for five minutes.
3. Blend with a hand blender, but save some of the mix before doing so and add to the soup pot after blending.

Fish and Noodle Soup (Serves 2)

Ingredients

½ packet soba, udon or rice noodles
2 pieces of boneless fish
1 tablespoon fish sauce
1 tablespoon sesame (preferably toasted) oil
Sea salt and black pepper to taste
2 cups vegetable stock
2 tablespoons miso paste

Toppings: green onion (side cut), coriander leaves, lime wedges, ground peanut, red spicy chutney

Method

1. Boil vegetable stock.
2. Prepare noodles separately.
3. Heat the oil in a skillet. Add fish, fish sauce and stir-fry for 2–3 minutes. Season with salt and pepper.
4. Divide noodles between two bowls, first put the fish on top, then pour the stock.
5. Mix in the miso paste.
6. Top up the dish with your selection of toppings.

Probiotic Pumpkin Soup (Serves 2)

Ingredients

250g red pumpkin (bhopla/lal kaddu)
1 onion, diced

½ carrot, cubed
A pinch of cinnamon
Sea salt to taste
2 tablespoons miso paste
Parsley for garnishing

Method

1. Boil pumpkin, carrots and onions together in a cup of water.
2. Add cinnamon and sea salt.
3. Once done, blend with a hand blender.
4. Add miso paste.
5. Garnish with parsley before serving.

Lentil Soup (Serves 2)

Ingredients

½ cup yellow lentils (pigeon pea [toovar] or channa [gram])
½ teaspoon cumin seeds
½ teaspoon turmeric
½ teaspoon red chilli flakes
1 cup vegetable stock
1 teaspoon cardamom seeds
1 teaspoon mustard seeds
½ onion, sliced into half moons
1 garlic pod, crushed
1 teaspoon white miso
Sea salt to taste

Method

1. Pressure-cook lentils in vegetable stock, cumin and chilli flakes, and purée once done.
2. Heat oil in a pan, add mustard and cardamom seeds, and fry till they pop. Then add the onion and garlic, and cook till it browns a bit. Then, add turmeric powder.
3. Mix in with the lentils and give it a stir.
4. Once lentil soup is ready, add the miso paste or sea salt to taste.

Cold Soups

These soups can be used when you are doing a detox in March (spring). It can be used as a starter at lunch or dinner.

Good-Gut Gazpacho (Serves 6)

Ingredients

4 cups tomato juice
½ cup finely minced onion
1 medium clove of garlic, minced
1 medium bell pepper, minced
1 teaspoon honey (optional)
1 medium cucumber, peeled, seeded and minced
Juice of 1 lime
1 teaspoon basil
1–1½ teaspoon cumin powder
¼ cup minced coriander

2–3 tablespoons olive oil
2 cups diced tomatoes
3 tablespoons white miso paste
Salt, black pepper and red chilli powder to taste

Method

Combine all ingredients (or purée them). Chill until very cold.

Chilled Cucumber Yogurt Soup (Serves 4–6)

Ingredients

4 cups peeled, seeded and grated cucumber
2 cups water
2 cups yogurt (non-dairy preferably)
½–1 teaspoon salt
1 small clove of garlic, minced
1 teaspoon dried dill (or 1 tablespoon fresh dill)
1 tablespoon honey (optional)
Minced fresh mint

Method

1. Combine grated cucumber, water, yogurt, salt, garlic, dill, and honey (optional) in a medium-sized bowl.
2. Stir until it is well blended, and chill until very cold.
3. Serve topped with finely minced fresh mint.

Almost Kefir Chilled Berry Soup (Serves 4–6)

Ingredients

> 3 cups orange juice
> 3 cups buttermilk or yogurt (non-dairy preferred)
> 1–2 tablespoons fresh lemon or lime juice
> 1–2 tablespoons honey (optional)
> 2–3 cups berries in any combination (add smaller berries as it is; larger ones should be sliced)
> A dash of cinnamon and/or nutmeg and a few sprigs of fresh mint for garnish (optional)

Method

1. Whisk together orange juice and buttermilk or yogurt. Add lemon or lime juice and honey (optional) to taste. Cover and chill until serving time.
2. When you are ready to serve, place about ½ cup of berries in each bowl. Ladle the soup on top. If desired, dust very lightly with cinnamon and/ or nutmeg, and garnish with a few small sprigs of mint.

Grains in Another Way!

Bacteria-Boosting Brown-Rice Salad (Servings: 4)

This makes for a great meal to carry to work or when you are on the run. It's complete with vegetables and can be had cold.

Ingredients

2 cups cooked basic brown rice
3 cups boiling water
1 small onion, diced
6 green beans, cut diagonally
1 cup cabbage, 1-inch pieces or cut fine
1 cup carrot, small cubes
2 onions, cut small
4 tablespoons sunflower seeds (optional)
½ cup chopped sauerkraut
Basic vinaigrette dressing (blend together 2 tablespoons olive oil and 1 tablespoon white wine vinegar or lime juice. Add ½ teaspoon mustard powder and salt to taste)

Method

1. Add beans, carrot and onion to boiling water. Do not overboil the vegetables; they should be crisp.
2. Retain water as you lift the vegetables out with a strainer.
3. Blanch cabbage in the same boiling water for just 1 minute.
4. You can reuse this broth if you want in a soup.
5. Mix all the other ingredients and use a basic vinaigrette dressing.

Brown-Rice Croquettes (Servings: 6 croquettes)

Ingredients

3 cups of cooked basic brown rice
1 carrot, grated
1 onion, cut small and fine
3 cloves of garlic, chopped fine
3 tablespoons black sesame seeds, roasted
½ cup whole grain breadcrumbs
½ cup coriander leaves
1 tablespoon extra virgin olive oil
Sea salt, a little chilli powder or black pepper powder

Method

1. Add oil and sauté carrot, onion and garlic in a pan on a low fire, and keep it covered for five minutes.
2. Mix in with the rice.
3. Add dry spices and coriander leaves.
4. Shape into 8 croquettes (you can wet your hands with water while doing this).
5. Mix breadcrumbs and black sesame seeds on a plate.
6. Roll the croquettes so they are coated on both sides.
7. Pan-fry in a shallow dish or bake at 150 degrees Celsius for forty minutes on a foil sheet that is oiled.

Barley and Mushroom Risotto (Serves 8)

Ingredients

1 cup pearl barley
1 tablespoon ghee
1⅓ cup onions, chopped
8 shiitake mushrooms, soaked overnight and stem removed in the morning, sliced long
½ cup regular button mushrooms, chopped fine
1 tablespoon garlic, chopped
6 cups vegetable stock
Sea salt and black pepper to taste

Method

1. To a skillet, add ghee, onions and garlic, and cook till translucent.
2. Add the button mushrooms first, cover and cook till tender.
3. Once tender, add some water and cook a little longer.
4. Use a hand blender to blend the mushrooms to a grainy texture (this provides the creamy base for the risotto).
5. Add the shiitake mushrooms and sauté for a while on medium heat.
6. Add the pearl barley and sauté for at least four minutes. Combine the salt and pepper.

7. Add the vegetable stock and let it boil, covered, for forty-five minutes till barley is done.

Quiet-Stomach Quinoa Pilaf (Serves 2)

Ingredients

½ cup quinoa, rinsed well
1 cup water or vegetable stock
1–2 garlic pods, minced
1 medium onion, sliced thinly
1 red bell pepper, seeded and roasted with skin removed, and diced
½ teaspoon each of turmeric, cumin (jeera) powder and coriander (dhaniya) powder
½ cup cooked chickpeas (optional)
Cardamom (*elaichi*) powder
1 fistful coriander leaves
1 fistful mint leaves
1 tablespoon olive oil
Sea salt and pepper to taste

Method

1. Add quinoa to boiling water or vegetable stock. Cover and simmer till done.
2. Add oil to a frying pan or skillet. Add onions, garlic, red bell pepper and chickpeas. Cook for about 3–4 minutes, and then add the dry spices.

3. Add quinoa to this veggie mix. Season with sea salt and pepper.
4. Stir in coriander and mint before serving.

Fibre-Full Foxtail Millet (Cheena) with Vegetables (Serves 4)

This can be used as a salad or pilaf.

Ingredients

½ carrot, cut into cubes
1 cup cooked millet
½ cup chopped celery
1 tablespoon lemon zest
2 tablespoons chopped mint
2 tablespoons chopped coriander
¼ cup sauerkraut

For Dressing

¼ cup olive oil
2 teaspoons ground cumin
1 teaspoon turmeric
3 tablespoons lemon juice
Sea salt and pepper to taste
Whisk the above ingredients in a small blender.

Method

1. Fluff the cooked millet with a fork or use hands to smear olive oil and rub in the millet so as not to form lumps.
2. Stir in the celery, mint, coriander, carrots, lemon zest and mix well. Then add sauerkraut.
3. Pour the dressing over the top.

MAC-Rich Mint Couscous with Vegetables (Serves 4)

Ingredients

1 carrot, cut into big chunks
1 turnip (shalgam), cut into quarters
1 zucchini, cut into 2-inch pieces
½ sweet potato, cut into chunks
2 tomatoes, skin removed and chopped
2 tablespoons tomato paste (puréed in a blender)
1½ cups vegetable stock
1 tablespoon olive oil
2–3 garlic cloves, minced
1 tablespoon chilli powder
1 teaspoon cumin powder
½ teaspoon ginger, crushed
1 green chilli (optional)
1 bay leaf (tej patta)
½ cup chopped sauerkraut
Sea salt and black pepper to taste

Method

1. Pre-boil vegetables (you can pressure-cook the turnip so that they get done faster).
2. Warm oil in a wok, add garlic and dry spices, and cook for 1–2 minutes. Add tomato paste and chopped tomatoes.
3. Add vegetable stock and bring to a boil.
4. Then add the vegetables and season with sea salt and pepper.
5. In a separate pan, make the couscous and add the mint after it's done. Then cover with a cling wrap and keep covered till your vegetables get ready.
6. Open it up and fluff with a fork. Add the sea salt and pepper if required, pour the vegetable mix over the couscous and serve warm.
7. Add sauerkraut.

Fusilli Salad (Serves 4)

Ingredients

300g dried wholewheat fusilli (try using gluten-free, if possible)
150g green beans, cut in 1-inch pieces
1 small avocado, diced
1 red bell pepper, roasted, skinned and diced
400g white soy beans cooked and drained
4–5 mounaka raisins, seeded

For Dressing

2 teaspoons curry powder
1 teaspoon cumin
8 tablespoons soy yogurt
8 tablespoons tofu mayonnaise
3 tablespoons lime juice
Sea salt and black pepper
Whisk all ingredients in a blender together to form a thick creamy dressing.

Method

1. Cook fusilli in boiling water till it is al dente.
2. Blanch green beans in boiling water for five minutes.
3. Put together cooked fusilli, green beans, soy beans, avocado and toss in the raisins and bell pepper.
4. Add dressing and chill before serving.

Tabbouleh-Style Quinoa (Serves 2)

Ingredients

½ cup quinoa
2 green onions, cut sideways (like you see in Chinese food)
1 tomato
½ cup boiled peas
A fistful of parsley
A fistful of coriander
2 tablespoons walnuts (optional)
¼ cup sauerkraut

For Dressing

> 3 tablespoons extra virgin olive oil
> 1 teaspoon Dijon mustard
> 2 garlic pods, crushed
> Juice of ½ lime
> Sea salt and black pepper to taste

Method

1. Prepare quinoa by rinsing thoroughly and boiling in 1 cup of water.
2. Chop the onion and tomato.
3. When quinoa is done, add the chopped vegetables, peas, coriander and parsley.
4. Mix together gently.
5. Mix in salad dressing.
6. Toast walnuts in a pan, chop roughly (after cooling) and toss into the quinoa.
7. Toss in sauerkraut.

Salads

Radish, Red Grape and Rocket/Arugula Leaf Salad (Serves 4–6)

Ingredients

> 1 bunch of arugula, rinsed and well-trimmed
> 1 cucumber, peeled and diced

2 ripe tomatoes, diced

4–5 radishes, diced

2–3 green onions, thinly sliced diagonally

2–3 cups red grapes, halved

½ cup sauerkraut

For Dressing

½ cup sesame seeds, roasted

2–3 red onions, diced

½ cup extra virgin olive oil

3 tablespoons balsamic vinegar

2 tablespoons red wine vinegar

Sea salt

Blend the ingredients in a small blender and pour olive oil in a steady stream from the top.

Method

1. Keep the arugula leaves in chilled ice water.
2. Combine all vegetables and fruit in a bowl, and toss in the dressing (save some for arugula leaves).
3. Remove arugula from water, wipe with a clean cloth and toss in the dressing.
4. Plate the leaves first and mound the vegetables on the top.
5. Toss in the sauerkraut.

Stomach-Friendly Squash Salad (Serves 2)

Ingredients

250g red pumpkin (bhopla/lal kaddu) cut into half rounds
4 pods of garlic, chopped fine
4 tablespoons balsamic vinegar
2 teaspoons basil
A bunch of arugula
2 tablespoons olive oil

Method

1. Parboil the squash.
2. Set your oven to 200 degrees Celsius.
3. Sauté garlic and basil in olive oil.
4. Add the squash and toss till coated.
5. Bake for twenty minutes until slightly brown.
6. Remove arugula from the chilled water, wipe with a clean towel.
7. Toss it in 1 tablespoon of balsamic vinegar and ½ teaspoon of olive oil.
8. Put the arugula on a plate (which is the base of this salad).
9. Layer the squash on the top to serve.

Microbiota-Rich Marinated Bell Peppers (Serves 6)

Ingredients

6 medium-sized bell peppers of different colours (de-skin the red peppers)
2 tablespoons olive oil
½–1 teaspoon basil
½ teaspoon marjoram or oregano
2 medium-sized garlic, minced
1–2 tablespoons red wine vinegar
Fresh black pepper and salt to taste

Method

1. Steam and seed the bell peppers, and cut into strips.
2. Heat olive oil in a skillet. Add bell peppers, salt, herbs and black pepper. Cook, stirring over medium heat for about five minutes and then add garlic. Sauté another few minutes, or until the peppers are tender.
3. Remove from heat and immediately stir in the vinegar. Let it marinate at room temperature for at least an hour. Store in refrigerator tightly covered. Serve at any temperature.

Prebiotic-Powered Sweet Potatoes and Broccoli (Serves 6)

Ingredients

3 medium-sized sweet potatoes
1 large broccoli floret
Toasted walnuts for garnish

For Marinade

½ cup olive oil
1 large garlic clove, minced
3 tablespoons lemon juice
2 tablespoons red wine vinegar
1 teaspoon sea salt
1 tablespoon dry mustard
1 tablespoon honey
Freshly ground black pepper

Method

1. Cut sweet potatoes into quarters and slice thin, and cook in boiling water.
2. Combine marinade ingredients in a small mixing bowl.
3. Add warm sweet potato slices to the marinade and mix gently.
4. Steam broccoli until bright green and tender. Rinse under cold water and drain.
5. Lay broccoli spears on top of the potatoes and mix together. Cover in a cling wrap and refrigerate for several hours.
6. Garnish with toasted walnuts while serving.

Organism-Fuelled Odessa Beet Salad (Serves 6)

Ingredients

5–6 medium beets, pressure-cooked and grated
2–3 tablespoons lemon juice

8–10 mounaka raisins, seeded
2–3 medium garlic cloves, minced
½ teaspoon sea salt
½ cup walnuts, toasted
1 cup chopped pineapple, cubed
½ cup sauerkraut

Method

1. Mix all ingredients together.
2. Chill until serving and toss in the sauerkraut.

L-Glutamine-Rich Two-Tone Coleslaw (Serves 4)

Ingredients

225g green cabbage
225g red cabbage
1 carrot
1 apple
½ cup mounaka, seeded

For Dressing

Use green earth dip

Method

1. Slice or shred cabbage into thin strips.
2. Mix all ingredients with the green earth dip.

Greens Salad (Serves 4)

Ingredients

Any leafy greens, about 8–10 leaves
1 tablespoon red wine vinegar
1 tablespoon shallots (what Indians call Madras onions)
½ teaspoon mustard
Sea salt and black pepper
Walnuts (optional)
½ cup sauerkraut

Method

1. Whisk together the red vinegar, shallots, mustard, sea salt and black pepper.
2. Toss in the greens.
3. Add walnuts at the end (optional).
4. Toss in the sauerkraut.

Carrot Mung Bean Salad (Serves 4)

Ingredients

¼ cup green mung, soaked overnight and boiled
1 large carrot, grated
½ red bell pepper, skinned and diced
1 teaspoon ginger, grated
2 tablespoons lemon juice
½ teaspoon mustard seeds
1 small green chilli, chopped

10 curry leaves
1 tablespoon coriander leaves
Salt to taste

Method

1. Heat oil in a skillet, add mustard seeds and let them pop. When popping stops, add chilli and curry leaves, and fry for 30 seconds.
2. Add this to a mixture of green mung, carrots, bell pepper and ginger. Then add coriander leaves and lemon juice.
3. Add salt and toss gently before serving.

Power-Protein Tofu Salad (Serves 2)

This is great in a sandwich, on crackers or by itself. It can be used at breakfast to substitute your egg consumption. While bringing in a great source of digestible protein and giving you the B vitamins, minerals, phosphorus, iron, sodium, potassium and low calories (18 calories per ounce), tofu also has the calcium content equal to that of milk.

Ingredients

1 pack of silken Mori-Nu tofu or any other tofu (8 ounces)
1 onion, grated
2 celery stalks, cut fine
2 carrots, grated
1 tablespoon white wine vinegar
Sea salt to taste

Method

1. Steam the tofu (make sure all the water is squeezed out of your tofu block) and keep aside.
2. Mix all the other ingredients. Crumble tofu with your hand and mix well.
3. Chill for 10–15 minutes before serving.

Beans

Refried Beans (Serves 6–8)

Ingredients

2 cups cooked red kidney beans (*rajma*), mashed when warm
2–3 tablespoons olive oil
2 cups onions, minced
5–6 garlic pods, minced
1–2 teaspoons sea salt
Black pepper
1 small green bell pepper, minced
1 tablespoon cumin powder

Method

1. Heat olive oil in a skillet. Add onions, garlic, cumin and salt, and sauté for 5–7 minutes till onions are pink.
2. Add bell pepper and black pepper.
3. Turn heat to low and add cooked beans.

4. Cook for about ten minutes till all flavours are absorbed.

Red Kidney Bean Cutlets (Serves 4)

Ingredients

2 tablespoons canola oil
1 small red bell pepper, seeded and chopped small
½ cup celery, chopped
1 large garlic clove, minced
½ teaspoon chilli powder
½ teaspoon dried thyme
Sea salt and fresh ground black pepper
1½ cups cooked red kidney beans
½ cup cooked brown rice
½ cup breadcrumbs
2 tablespoons parsley

Method

1. Heat oil and add all ingredients, except salt and pepper. Cover and cook, stirring occasionally until soft (about ten minutes).
2. In a food processor, combine everything and add salt and pepper, and process it all together.
3. Pulse, without grinding it entirely and leaving some texture.
4. Shape into patties and set aside; you can add breadcrumbs to bind them.
5. Pan-fry patties on both sides till brown.

Antioxidant-Rich Chickpea Peppery Salad (Serves 4)

Ingredients

1 onion, diced
1 each of red, yellow and green bell pepper, diced (remove skin of red pepper)
2 cups cooked chickpeas
2 bundles bok choy, cut long and steamed
Olives (optional)

For Dressing

¼ cup olive oil
3 tablespoons balsamic vinegar
3 garlic cloves, minced
Grated zest of 1 lime and juice
Sea salt to taste

Method

Put together ingredients in a salad bowl and toss.

Divine Burrito with Black Beans (Serves 6)

Ingredients

1 cup brown rice, cooked
2 tablespoons extra virgin olive oil
1 yellow bell pepper, seeded and cut into strips
1 red bell pepper, roasted, seeded and cut into strips

1 onion, sliced into half moons
1 tablespoon chilli powder
2 teaspoons cumin powder
½ teaspoon sea salt
½ kg tomatoes, roasted and chopped
2 cups black beans, cooked
6 tortillas
Some avocado and salsa
½ cup chopped sauerkraut

Method

1. Heat olive oil in a pan, sauté peppers and onions for about seven minutes.
2. Add dry spices and sauté for about ten minutes.
3. Add tomatoes, lower heat and cook for seven minutes.
4. Pour into a bowl and add beans and rice. Stir well.
5. To make burritos, heat tortillas until warm. Add 1 big spoonful of peppers and onion mixture. Then layer with avocado and salsa. Add sauerkraut.
6. Roll and serve.

Stir-Fry Tofu and Black Bean (Serves 2)

Ingredients

½ cup black kidney beans (rajma)
8 ounces of tofu, cubed
Small piece (½ inch) of ginger, sliced long

1–2 garlic cloves, minced
2 tablespoons corn, boiled
1 teaspoon toasted sesame oil
2 green onions, cut sideways
Sea salt and black pepper

Method

1. Soak black beans overnight and pressure-cook the next day.
2. Heat the oil in wok and add tofu. Fry both sides and set aside.
3. Add ginger and garlic to the same wok.
4. Add the black beans and corn, and stir-fry for five minutes on a high flame.
5. Add tofu and cook for 2–3 minutes.
6. Season with sea salt and pepper.
7. Garnish with spring onions.

Fish

Flavourful Soba Noodles with Fish and Vegetables (Serves 2)

Ingredients

100g of soba noodles (buckwheat), cooked in hot water
1 fish fillet, pan-fried or steamed

1–2 cups vegetable stock
½–1 tablespoon soy sauce
1-inch piece ginger, cut into strips
2 green onions, side-cut
1 red bell pepper, seeded and skinned (post-roasting), cut into strips
1 carrot, cut thin-finger size
3–4 pieces of bamboo shoots, cut into strips
4 bok choy leaves, cut into strips
1 teaspoon toasted sesame oil
Fistful of coriander leaves
Sea salt to taste or miso (1 teaspoon)
1 tablespoon kudzu to thicken the sauce

Method

1. Pan-fry or steam fish, after brushing some oil over it.
2. Boil vegetable stock, add soy sauce, ginger and all the vegetables and bring to a boil. Reduce heat and simmer for five minutes.
3. Add toasted sesame oil.
4. You can mix 1 tablespoon of kudzu in cool water (½ cup) and add to this sauce to thicken it.
5. Add miso or sea salt at this point.
6. Divide noodles and pour the vegetable broth over the noodles. Place the fish on top.
7. Garnish with coriander leaves.

Fats-Galore Fish Burgers (Serves 4)

Ingredients

2 fillets of any fish, steamed
½ cup regular flour
½ cup breadcrumbs
Sea salt, black pepper and a dash of mustard
½ cup chopped sauerkraut
4 tablespoons tofu mayonnaise

For Fillers

Cucumber, sliced
Tomato, sliced
Lettuce, sliced

Method

1. In a bowl, combine fish, flour and breadcrumbs with sea salt, pepper and mustard.
2. Shape into burger croquettes.
3. Pan-fry in a non-stick frying pan.
4. Assemble the burgers by first toasting the buns and spreading tofu mayonnaise on them. Then layer the lettuce, cucumber, fish burger patty, tomatoes and sauerkraut.

Steamed Fish (Serves 2)

Ingredients

2 pieces of basa or any other fish

Juice of 1 lime
1 tablespoon olive oil
1 tablespoon garlic and ginger paste
Sea salt and black pepper

Method

1. Take a knife and make thin cuts on the fish fillets or steaks.
2. Mix all the above ingredients and smear on both sides of fish.
3. Keep in the fridge for about two hours.
4. Steam before you want to eat the fish for about seven minutes.

Asian Salmon with Brown Rice (Serves 2)

Ingredients

½–1-inch piece ginger
2 garlic cloves, minced
½ carrot, sliced thinly
2½ cups mushrooms, sliced
2 tablespoons coriander, chopped
2 teaspoons honey
2 salmon fish steaks (if you don't get salmon, please use any other fish)
1 cup cooked brown rice
1 teaspoon Chinese five-spice powder
1 tablespoon soy sauce
Sea salt and white pepper to taste

For Chinese Five-Spice Powder

1 teaspoon pepper (Schezwan pepper preferred)
1 teaspoon ground star anise
1 teaspoon ground fennel seeds
½ teaspoon ground cloves
½ teaspoon ground cinnamon
½ teaspoon sea salt
¼ teaspoon white pepper
Combine all the ingredients after dry-roasting and grind together (optional) or let it stay whole.

Method

1. Marinate the fish (after washing) in the Chinese five-spice powder, by smearing on either side of the fish steaks.
2. Steam or broil the fish steaks for ten minutes.
3. Heat a pan and add soy sauce, ginger, garlic, honey and carrots. Warm it for 4–5 minutes until the mixture softens. Add mushrooms and sauté for 2–3 minutes.
4. Season with sea salt and white pepper.
5. Plate warm brown rice. Add vegetables and fish on top.
6. Garnish with chopped coriander.

Note: You can chop mushrooms and sauté with tomatoes to change flavour and add variety.

Fermented Foods

Probiotic-Rich Pressed Salad (Servings: 4)

This is a great source of vitamin B12 for vegetarians and vegans.

Ingredients

½ cup sliced cucumbers
½ cup sliced cabbage
½ cup red radish
¼ cup celery
¼ cup red onion
1 teaspoon salt

Note: Adding green apples, when in season, make this salad nice and tangy.

Method

1. Mix all the vegetables with sea salt in a large bowl, and gently press and mix with fingers until they wilt.
2. Place a plate on top of the vegetables and press down with a heavy weight. I usually have a brick that I have kept handy, wrapped in a clean cloth. You can also use a vessel filled with water to put on the plate.
3. Allow it to stand for forty-five minutes; let the water drain out from the vegetables.
4. Discard or drink the water (it is full of probiotic bacteria). Rinse with fresh filter water if you find it too salty to drink.
5. Eat as a side dish.

Note: The breakdown of sugars in the vegetables and the process of lacto-fermentation that takes place cause the good bacteria to come in, therefore making this dish the perfect fermented food to use daily by varying the vegetables.

Pressed salad will help assimilate your entire meal and provide quick fermentation and good bacteria. You can even save some and have it the next day with another meal. I highly recommend this dish if you want to do a three-day detox.

Papaya Khimchi (Makes 1 large 500g bottle)

Ingredients

1 medium-sized green papaya (approximately 1½kg), peeled, seeded and julienned or shredded
½ red bell pepper, burnt, made to sweat, skin removed and sliced long
1 medium carrot, shredded
1½-inch-piece ginger, sliced thin
2–3 garlic pods, sliced thin
1½ cups apple cider vinegar
½ cup sugar substitute (like stevia)
2 tablespoons sea salt
½ cup pineapple juice

Method

1. Squeeze the papaya juice and put the papaya in a flat dish. Spread and dry in the sun for one hour.

2. Combine vinegar, sugar substitute and salt in a small saucepan and simmer till everything dissolves.
3. Add pineapple juice and mix well.
4. In the same flat dish (in which papaya is kept to dry), combine the rest of the vegetables, including garlic and ginger, and add this liquid mixture. Press with a heavy substance, such as a brick wrapped in a towel or a large heavy dish, for one hour.
5. After one hour, this khimchi can be stored in the fridge for up to two weeks.

Beetroot Pickle (Makes 1 bottle of 250g)

Ingredients

250g beetroot, skinned and sliced thin
¼ teaspoon sea or rock salt
½ teaspoon of round cardamom (elaichi)

Method

1. Add sliced beetroot to a jar.
2. Dissolve the cardamom in warm water and add salt; pour over beetroot. Make sure the beetroot is submerged in water.
3. Once it tastes tangy and begins to get cloudy, put a lid on it and refrigerate.
4. Consume over the next few weeks.

Note: The same process can be used with apple cider vinegar (instead of water), but I would suggest using a mixture of water and apple cider vinegar in an equal ratio.

Turmeric Pickle (Makes 1 bottle)

Ingredients

250g raw haldi
1 cup apple cider vinegar (or brown rice vinegar)

Method

1. Slice haldi into slivers.
2. Add vinegar to a bottle and then the haldi.
3. Tie the mouth with a muslin cloth or handkerchief.
4. Leave in the sun for three days.
5. Refrigerate.

Carrot Kanji (Servings: 8–10)

Ingredients

5 medium-sized carrots
2 small beetroots
8 cups of water (boiled and filtered)
1–1½ teaspoons red chilli powder
Black salt
2 tablespoons mustard powder (dry-ground)

Method

1. Rinse and skin carrots and beetroot. Cut them into long slices.
2. Mix all the ingredients in a glass or ceramic jar.

3. Cover with a muslin cloth and keep it in the sun for 3–4 days.
4. Stir the mixture with a wooden spoon every day and keep the jar back in the sun.
5. When it starts tasting sour, it means it's ready.
6. Refrigerate.

Rejuvelac (Servings 4–6)

Ingredients

One cup soft wheat berries

Note: You can also use rye, quinoa, buckwheat or other grains. Wheat, rye and quinoa seem to make the best rejuvelac.

Method

1. Place the wheat berries in a sprouting jar (1 litre) with a screen top and fill with water.
2. Soak the grain for twenty-four hours. Drain off water, leave berries in jar and rinse two to three times a day until little sprout tails appear.
3. Place the sprouted grain in a large jar with a top that allows air to circulate. Add 4 cups of water and let it sit on the counter for 2–3 days.
4. You will notice the water getting cloudy and little bubbles forming.
5. It should taste clean and fresh, with a hint of lemon flavour. Strain the rejuvelac and store in a covered

glass container in the refrigerator. Keep it there for at least a week. Just make sure it still smells and tastes fresh. You can reuse the wheat berries to make a second batch. It will only take a day.

Note: Since some people may have a hard time adjusting to the taste, you can add some tea bags or ginger and lime juice (at room temperature) to the rejuvelac to make it drinkable.

Pickled Ginger (Makes 1 bottle of 250g)

Ingredients

250g ginger, peeled and sliced thin
1 teaspoon cloves
¼ teaspoon rock/sea salt

Method

1. Fill a small bottle with warm water.
2. Add cloves and salt, and dissolve it.
3. Add ginger, leaving an inch from the mouth of the jar, but make sure it is submerged in water.
4. Cover with a muslin cloth and leave in the sun or kitchen counter for 3–5 days.
5. When it seems cloudy and tastes tangy, cover the lid and refrigerate.
6. It can be used over the next 3–4 weeks.

Note: The same process can be done using apple cider vinegar as well. There are two more good vinegars called ume sho kudzu (made with the wondrous ume plum) and brown rice vinegar (see Source List).

Sauerkraut (For a 500g bottle)

Traditionally, sauerkraut is made from finely cut cabbage fermented by lactic acid bacteria. It means 'sour cabbage' in German. It was known to provide all the nutrients when consumed in a small quantity in colder climates, when transportation of foods was difficult from warmer climates. Fermentation by lactobacilli is introduced naturally, when salt is added to the cabbage as the bacteria in the air start breaking down the sugars in the cabbage. You don't have to use cabbage; you can use any other hardy vegetables like beetroot, carrots, radish, finely cut cucumber or green peppers.

It is important to keep your workspace clean when making sauerkraut; this includes the dishes used to make them.

Ingredients

12 cups of shredded cabbage (approximately 1kg)
1 tablespoon sea/rock salt

Method (See Pictures)

1. Peel off the outer layer of cabbage, if discoloured.
2. Cut the cabbage lengthwise into four pieces.
3. Start chopping it fine (lengthwise); keep the sliced bits as uniform as possible.
4. Don't throw the core or the outer leaves (yet).

5. Put the cabbage in a large bowl.

6. Sprinkle salt into it.

7. Work the salt into the cabbage by tossing and turning it (this helps breakdown the cell walls and draw out water from the cabbage). This starts the fermentation process by creating lactic acid, which is the juice in which it will ferment eventually.

8. Do this for 5–10 minutes.

9. It will start to wilt and shrink.

10. When the cabbage has shrunk to half its original volume, you can taste it; it will be salty.

11. Now take a jar and start packing the cabbage into it (pack it tight, so as to leave no air between layers), till it is two inches below the mouth of the jar.

12. You can now use the outer leaves as a layer on the top to keep the cabbage down and the core as a weight on the top of the outer leaves (this will be at the mouth of the jar).

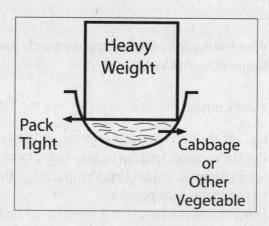

13. All the water (brine as we call it) should cover the cabbage; the cabbage should be submerged in the brine.

14. If you don't have enough brine, you can make some more by taking 1 cup of water at room temperature and adding 1 tablespoon salt.

15. Make sure there is some space between the brine and the outer rim of the jar (this is in case some carbon dioxide (which is generated during the fermentation process) pushes the cabbage upwards.

16. You can cover the jar with the lid, but it should not be tightly screwed. Cover it using a heavy weight pressing the cabbage down.

17. Set it aside in a dark space and do not keep it in the light.

18. Put a plate underneath in case the liquid brine bubbles out of the jar.

19. Make sure the cabbage is submerged in water. If not, make some brine and re-submerge it in the brine.

20. After a week, the sauerkraut is ready to be consumed.

21. Store it in the fridge to slow the fermentation process.

22. Always make sure the brine covers the vegetables used.

23. Do not heat the kraut ever, as bacteria die if heated over 43 degrees Celsius. So, if you add it to food such as rolls, wraps, grilled sandwiches, etc., make sure the food is cool.

Kraut Tips

(1) If you see mouldy kraut (discoloured or smelly), remove it from the main vegetables. This does not mean your kraut has gone bad; it may happen to your topmost leaves.

(2) The kraut could become sludgy and slimy-looking in a warmer climate or if not enough salt was used. Wait and watch. If it doesn't disappear, remove that bit from your kraut.

(3) You must tend to your kraut like you would a child, taking care of it and watching over it daily. It takes patience and practice. But in the end, it's worth the wait!

Sweet Potato Pickle (Serves 2)

Ingredients

2 tablespoons stevia powder and 1 tablespoon golden sugar (Conscious Foods)
4–5 limes
1 tablespoon chopped coriander leaves
3 Kashmiri chillies, chopped small
½kg potato, cubed small (boiled till they are still firm)
Rock or sea salt to taste

Method

1. Peel of skin of the limes and cut it length-wise into segments.
2. Leave segments as they are and add stevia and sugar.
3. Add chillies, salt and coriander leaves.
4. Add the above mix to sweet potato, leave on table top for an hour (cover with muslin cloth).
5. Refrigerate overnight, before using the next day.

Dressings/Sauces/Dips

Tofu Cream (Serves 6)

Ingredients

1 pack of Mori-Nu silken tofu or tofu that has a creamy consistency (you may have to add soy milk to get this)
2 tablespoons lemon juice
1 tablespoon miso (white)
2 teaspoons olive oil

Method

1. Steam tofu in a steamer for 3–5 minutes; let it cool a bit.
2. Add all the ingredients to it and whip together.

Note: Sometimes I add 1 teaspoon mustard to it to give it a twist (this is especially good for your liver).

Lemon Tahini Dressing (Serves 1)

Ingredients

2 tablespoons tahini
1 tablespoon lemon juice
1 teaspoon white miso (optional)
Water to achieve desired consistency

Method

1. Place tahini, lemon juice and miso (optional) in a small bowl and mix well.
2. Add 1 tablespoon water at a time and mix until the desired consistency is achieved.
3. Use immediately or cover and chill till ready to use.

Smooth and Sweet Veggie Carrot Butter (Serves 6)

Just one carrot has all the vitamin A you need for the day!

Ingredients

4 cups carrots, cubed
1 tablespoon arrowroot powder dissolved in ¼ cup water
2 tablespoons tahini (sesame butter) or roasted and ground sesame seeds (put them in your dry grinder)
¼ cup water
1 teaspoon white miso
Sea salt to taste

Method

1. Boil carrots with the salt and let them cool.
2. Use a blender to blend, using some liquid (you could use the liquid you have used to boil the carrots).
3. Mix in the arrowroot liquid and put it on the gas to heat.
4. Keep stirring till the arrowroot thickens it a bit.
5. Add the tahini or ground sesame seeds (tahini usually works better) and miso paste.

Tomato Salsa (Yields 1½–2 cups)

Ingredients

3 medium-sized ripe tomatoes
2 green onions, minced
2 garlic cloves, minced
1 handful of parsley, minced
A handful of coriander, minced
1 teaspoon lightly roasted cumin seeds (jeera)
1 teaspoon salt
1 tablespoon fresh lime juice
1 tablespoon olive oil
½ cup sauerkraut, chopped
Crushed red pepper to taste

Method

1. Blanch tomatoes for seven seconds and remove.

2. Pull off the skins and seed the tomatoes.
3. Dice them.
4. Combine everything in a bowl.
5. Cover tightly and chill.

Red Pepper and Nut Salsa (Serves 4)

Ingredients

2 tablespoons walnuts or almonds, chopped
1–2 cloves garlic, chopped fine
2 tablespoons vinegar (apple cider or brown rice vinegar)
2 red bell peppers
5 tablespoons olive oil
Salt and black pepper to taste

Method

1. Preheat oven to 180 degrees Celsius.
2. Cut the red peppers lengthwise and seed it. Toss olive oil (2 teaspoons) and salt. Bake on an oiled sheet for 20 minutes. Once done, remove and set aside to cool.
3. When cooled, mix in the chopped nuts, garlic, vinegar and remaining olive oil.
4. Add salt and pepper to taste.

Marinara Sauce (Serves 8)

Ingredients

2 tablespoons extra virgin olive oil
4 garlic cloves, minced
1 red onion, diced
¼ teaspoon red pepper flakes
1 teaspoon thyme
1 teaspoon oregano
1kg tomato, roasted and chopped
½ cup tomato paste
1 tablespoon balsamic vinegar
2 teaspoons honey
2 tablespoons fresh basil, chopped
Sea salt and black pepper to taste

Method

1. Heat olive oil in a deep pan.
2. Sauté onion and garlic for about seven minutes.
3. Add thyme, red pepper flakes, oregano and fresh basil.
4. Add tomato and tomato paste.
5. Reduce the heat and simmer for thirty minutes.
6. Add honey, balsamic vinegar, sea salt and black pepper. Simmer for 5–10 minutes.
7. This can be stored in the refrigerator for up to five days.

Good-Gut Fat Guacamole (Serves 6)

Ingredients

2 tablespoons lemon juice
2 medium-sized ripe avocados
2 garlic cloves, minced
½ teaspoon sea salt
¼ cup chopped sauerkraut

You could add the following to spice it up:

Chilli powder
Green or red bell pepper, chopped fine
½ teaspoon cumin powder
Cucumber, chopped fine

Method

Mix all ingredients together, cover and chill.

Bone Broths

Chicken Bone Broth (Serves 4–6 times)

Ingredients

2–3 chicken necks and feet (or carcass of roast chicken)
Garlic cloves, smashed
Carrots, cut into chunks
Onions, cut into chunks
Spinach

3 tablespoons apple cider vinegar
2 bay leaves
Sea salt and pepper
Water (three times the amount of chicken)

Method

1. Bone broths usually work in slow cookers, cooked over twenty-four hours. However, you can slow boil for 4–6 hours. Make enough so that you can save it for the next few days.
2. Cook all the ingredients together.
3. Once done, strain and keep only the broth.
4. It can also be frozen and used later or consumed over a couple of days.

Note: Adapted from *Eat Dirt* by Josh Axe.

Koi-Koku (Fish Bone Soup) (Servings: 4)

Ingredients

Any fish with bones and scales intact, chopped into 3-inch pieces
Add lotus root, chopped into matchsticks
1 tablespoon ginger juice
1 tablespoon miso paste
Chopped green onions

Method

1. Sauté lotus root in oil.

2. Add vegetable stock (can use twig tea called *bancha* from Capt. Pawan, see Source List).
3. Add fish with bones and scales.
4. Cover with heavy lid and after one boil, simmer slowly for two hours.
5. When cooked and pieces are tender, add ginger juice (1 tablespoon or to taste).
6. Add 1 tablespoon miso paste and garnish with chopped green onions.
7. You can save any leftover in fridge and have over three days or freeze.

The Detoxifiers

Nishime (Serves 2)

Nishime literally means waterless cooking. The mechanics of this style is similar to steam energy, providing you with warm yang energy in the abdomen region. Vegetables cook in their own juices and stabilize blood sugar levels as they discharge yin foods like soft dairy (ice cream, cheese). As I mentioned earlier, nishime works like an internal generator for energy, and gives you steady energy over time. I would suggest having it 2–3 times for any meal. I prescribe this style regularly to Katrina Kaif and Jacqueline Fernandez when they need energy.

Ingredients

1 carrot, cut into chunks
¼ cabbage, cut into wedges

1 onion, cut into wedges
¼ cup squash, cut into wedges or cubed
2–3-inch strip of kombu (optional)
Soy sauce, ginger juice or any seasoning you like

Method

1. Place kombu at the bottom of the pot.
2. Layer vegetables one on top of each other and add little water.
3. Cover the pot and bring to a boil over a medium flame.
4. Lower flame and cook for twenty minutes.
5. If water evaporates, you can add some more.
6. When vegetables get tender, add a few drops of soy sauce, ginger juice or any seasoning you like.
7. Replace the cover for five minutes.
8. Remove from gas and let it sit for five minutes before serving.

Gomashio (Yields ½ bottle)

Gomashio combines sea salt and sesame seeds. The combination of oil and minerals from the salt help your blood condition to stay more alkaline and also gives you the calcium you require.

Ingredients

8 level tablespoons sesame seeds (tan or black)
1½ teaspoons sea salt

Method

1. Wash the sesame seeds in a strainer and allow water to drain.
2. Dry-roast the seeds on a medium flame.
3. Transfer sea salt to a bowl in which you can pound them.
4. When seeds leave an aroma and start to pop, they are ready (keep stirring with a wooden spatula till this stage).
5. Add seeds to the grinder bowl and pound and mix in a steady circular motion until 80–85 per cent is done or use a dry grinder to coarsely grind the seeds and salt (just whizz it once).
6. Store in a glass jar.
7. To use it, sprinkle ½–1 teaspoon on food.

Sweet Vegetable Drink (Makes 2 servings)

Drink this whenever you can, preferably in late afternoons. Drink warm once a day for one month. This relaxes the stomach, body and muscles, and curtails sweet cravings.

Ingredients

Use equal amounts of onions, carrots, cabbage and sweet squash, finely chopped

Method

1. Boil vegetables in water (four times the volume of vegetables) for 2–3 minutes. Reduce the flame to low.

2. Cover and let it simmer for twenty minutes.
3. Strain the vegetables from the broth. You can use them later in soups or stew.
4. Drink the broth, either hot or at room temperature.

Apple Kudzu Drink (Serves 1)

Ingredients

1 heaped teaspoon kudzu
½ cup apple juice
½ cup water

Method

1. Add ½ cup water to ½ cup of apple juice (preferably freshly prepared, by squeezing a grated apple).
2. Boil this slowly with 1 teaspoon dissolved kudzu powder and stir regularly until the preparation thickens.

Ume Sho Kudzu (Serves 1)

Ingredients

1 heaped teaspoon kudzu powder
1¼ cup cold water
½ ume plum
2–3 drops of shoyu (soy sauce)

Method

1. Dissolve 1 teaspoon kudzu in 2–3 tablespoons of water.

2. Add 1 cup of cold water to dissolved kudzu and boil on low flame, stirring constantly with a wooden spoon till it becomes translucent.
3. Add pulp of ½ pitted ume plum and ground to paste. Reduce the heat as you do so.
4. Add 2–3 drops of shoyu. Simmer for 2–3 minutes.
5. Drink hot.

Turmeric Milk (Serves 2)

We have all heard of the famous haldi *ka doodh*. To make the vegan version, substitute milk for coconut milk.

Ingredients

1 cup coconut milk
1 cup water
1 tablespoon ghee or coconut oil
1 teaspoon turmeric
Stevia (1 pill if using oils, 2–3 drops if using drops and ½ sachet if using granules)

Method

1. In a saucepan, combine water and coconut milk. Warm for two minutes.
2. Stir in ghee, turmeric and stevia to taste.

SOURCE LIST

For miso paste, brown rice, ume vinegar, ume paste, kudzu, shoyu, high-quality green tea, kombu, wakame, sea vegetables, bancha twig tea and brown rice syrup (natural sweetener):

Wakaba Japanese Food Company
Khasra No. 345/1,
Village Sultanpur, Near M.G. Road,
Near Metro Pillar No. 28B,
New Delhi-110030.
Phone: 9873923036 (Captain Pawan), 01164635577 (shop)
Email: capt_sadhana@hotmail.com

For Vaiswanara Choornam, *aswajith* (combination of ashwagandha and shilajit) and Ayurvedic panchakarma treatments:

Dr Raveendran and Dr Keshavan
The Arya Vaidya Chikitsalayam,
136/7 Trichy Road,
Ramanathapuram, Coimbatore-641045.
Phone: 0422-2367200, 0422-2313188
Email: frontoffice@avpayurveda.com

For all the superfoods suggested in the book, such as apple cider vinegar, goji berries, maca powder, inulin powder, raw cacao, hemp protein, coconut butter and omega-3, 6 and 9, go to:

iHerb.com
Amazon.com
Organicindia.com
Naturallyyours.in
Goindiaorganic.com

For organic whole grains, beans, lentils and speciality products like shiitake mushrooms and organic eggs:

Nature's Basket (in all major metros): Conscious Foods and 24 Letter Mantra, and their own brand, Healthy Alternatives
Conscious Foods, Mumbai: 022-24934551, 022-24934552
Navdanya, Mumbai: 022-66790081

For craniosacral therapy:

Quanta
Contact: Zia Nath
Makani Centre, 35th Road, Khar East, Mumbai-400050
Phone: 022-26487184
www.quantacare.org

Shibani Sachdeva
Craniosacral therapist
Phone: 9821028854

For fermented products like kefir, kombucha, sauerkraut, kanji and khimchee:

Shonali Sabherwal
Phone: 9819035604
www.soulfoodshonali.com
Email: shonaalii@macrobioticsindia.com

ACKNOWLEDGEMENTS

I want to thank Milee, my editor, for having continuous faith in my work and always being encouraging. I thank my mentors Mona Schwartz and S.N. Goenka, for giving me the two pillars of detox in my life: the macrobiotic diet and vipassana. My deepest gratitude to Dr P.T. Keshavan, Dr Raveendran, Dr Roopa, Dr Tara, Dr Soumit and Dr Tanuja at the Arya Vaidya Chikitsalayam, for making me centred and grounded in the principles of Ayurveda. My teachers at Kushi Institute who continue to be the conscience for my work in the field of macrobiotics in India: Warren Kramer, Bettina Zumdick, Lucci Baranda, John Kozinski and Carry Wolfe. I am grateful to my loving mom—my best friend and my most ardent fan—for the unconditional love she has given me all my life. I am grateful to Jacqueline Fernandez for believing in my work, and sticking it out with me for so long. I thank my uncle, Shiv, who continues to guide me on writing. To my team at home (staff) and at work for their continued support, without whom I would not be able to do the work that I do. I would like to thank Dr Bharathi Chawathe for being there for me as a guide for the last ten years of my life. Dr Agarwal, for believing in what I do, and showing that diet can play a crucial role in changing the health of people. Dr Nozer Sheriar, for being a positive force on my path to well-being. Big thanks to Dr Divya Chabria, for supporting me on the path of healing with homeopathy. I am indebted to Rakesh and Rekha Jhunjhunwalla, Jerry and Om Arora for their support.

Heartfelt thanks to Mini Shastri for believing in my work and opening doors for me in Delhi. Special thanks to Sonya, who has been there for me like an angel for the past year, for making me laugh and being an amazing human being; I know we have a friendship that goes back to many lives. Without my friends and their support, I don't know where I would have been, so here's to Brian, Upma, Lynn, Ajay (who has given me so much of his work ethic), Dilshad, Nisha, Simeron, Rahul, Kajal, Julie, Sarang, Radha, Sunita, Sharmila, Sue, Dalip T. and Sanjana Banaik.

And last but not the least, my family—my father, for watching over me and talking to me through his music; Gulzar uncle, for taking on my father's mantle; my aunt, Santosh, for being divine; my sister, Shabana, for always playing devil's advocate; my brother, Vishal, for being positive and constantly reminding me of the wool we have been knitted from; Pooja, my sister-in-law, for being a good friend; and Poonam aunty, for being the same. Love to my four sweeties—Azaan, Zara, Bella and Angel—for bringing out the inner child in me (love and thanks to the souls of Dude Senior, Dude Junior, Joy, Tipsy and Brutus).

A thank you to my clients and the ones who are yet to come, whose lives I hope to touch with my work.

NOTES

PART ONE

1. Your Forgotten Organ

1. Raphael Kellman, *The Microbiome Diet: The Scientifically Proven Way to Restore Your Gut Health and Achieve Permanent Weight Loss* (Boston: Da Capo Lifelong Books, 2014), 7.
2. Rob Knight, *Follow Your Gut* (New York: Simon & Schuster, 2015), 9.
3. Louis Pasteur, *Oeuvres de Pasteur* 3 (1857): 101.
4. Justin Sonnenberg and Erica Sonnenberg, *The Good Gut* (London: Penguin Press, 2015), 25.
5. Raphael Kellman, *The Microbiome Diet: The Scientifically Proven Way to Restore Your Gut Health and Achieve Permanent Weight Loss* (Boston: Da Capo Lifelong Books, 2014), 28.
6. Raphael Kellman, *The Microbiome Diet: the scientifically way to restore your gut health and achieve permanent weight loss,* (Da Capo Lifelong Books, 2014), p. 33
7. Knight, *Follow Your Gut,* 35.

8. Dr Josh Axe, *Eat Dirt: Why Leaky Gut May Be the Root Cause of Your Health Problems and 5 Surprising Steps to Cure It* (New York: HarperCollins, 2016), location 1150.

2. Leaky Gut and Inflammation

1. Hari Sharma, 'Ayurvedic Perspectives: Leaky Gut Syndrome, Dysbiosis, Ama, Free Radicals, and Natural Antioxidants', *An International Quarterly Journal of Research in Ayurveda* 30(2009): 90.
2. Dr Josh Axe, *Eat Dirt: Why Leaky Gut May Be the Root Cause of Your Health Problems and 5 Surprising Steps to Cure It* (New York: HarperCollins, 2016), location 839.
3. Dr David Perlmutter with Kristin Loberg, *Brain Maker: The Power of Gut Microbes to Heal and Protect Your Brain for Life* (London: Hachette, 2015), 56.
4. Justin Sonnenberg and Erica Sonnenberg, *The Good Gut* (London: Penguin Press, 2015), 62.
5. Raphael Kellman, *The Microbiome Diet: The Scientifically Proven Way to Restore Your Gut Health and Achieve Permanent Weight Loss* (Boston: Da Capo Lifelong Books, 2014), 39.
6. Mary Roach, *Gulp: Adventures on the Alimentary Canal* (London: Oneworld Publications, 2013), 120.
7. Sonnenberg and Sonnenberg, *The Good Gut,* 17.
8. 'Why getting more fibre in our diets is important', *Indian Express* (11 May 2015).

3. Your Microbes and Disease

1. 'Diet induced obesity is linked to marked but reversible alterations in the mouse distal gut microbiome', *Cell Host*

& *Microbe* 3 (2008): 212–23, in Knight, *Follow Your Gut,* 45.

2. Raphael Kellman, *The Microbiome Diet: The Scientifically Proven Way to Restore Your Gut Health and Achieve Permanent Weight Loss* (Boston: Da Capo Lifelong Books, 2014), 21.

3. Gerard E. Mullin, MD, *The Gut Balance Revolution* (Emmaus, PA: Rodale Books, 2015), location 297.

4. Judith Campisi, 'Aging, Cellular Senescence and Cancer', *Annual Reviews Physiology* 75 (2013): 685–705.

5. Nigma Talib, *Reverse the Signs of Ageing: The Revolutionary Inside-Out Plan to Glowing, Youthful Skin,* (London: Vermillion, 2015), 8.

6. Dr Josh Axe, *Eat Dirt: Why Leaky Gut May Be the Root Cause of Your Health Problems and 5 Surprising Steps to Cure It* (New York: HarperCollins, 2016), 205.

7. Mary Roach, *Gulp: Adventures on the Alimentary Canal* (London: Oneworld Publications, 2013), 303.

8. Rob Knight, *Follow Your Gut* (New York: Simon & Schuster, 2015), 46.

9. Axe, *Eat Dirt,* 404.

10. Sylvia M. Ferolla, Geyza N.A., Armiliato Claudia A. Couto and Teresa C.A. Ferrari, 'The role of intestinal bacteria overgrowth in obesity-related nonalcoholic fatty liver disease', *Nutrients* 6 (2014): 5584.

11. Dr David Perlmutter with Kristin Loberg, *Brain Maker: The Power of Gut Microbes to Heal and Protect Your Brain for Life* (London: Hachette, 2015), 56.

12. Dacher Keltner, *On The Vagus Nerve,* www.youtube.com/watch?v=5d6e_Un6dv8.

13. Perlmutter, *The Power of Gut Microbes,* 29.

14. Perlmutter, *The Power of Gut Microbes,* 47.

15. Dr David Perlmutter with Kristin Loberg, *Grain Brain* (London: Yellow Kite Books, 2014).

4. Food for the Microbiota to Flourish

1. Justin Sonnenberg and Erica Sonnenberg, *The Good Gut* (London: Penguin Press, 2015), 112.
2. Justin Sonnenberg and Erica Sonnenberg, *The Good Gut* (London: Penguin Press, 2015), 128.

PART TWO

7. Clean

1. Dr Mark Hyman, *Eat Fat, Get Thin* (Boston: Little, Brown and Company, 2016), 145.
2. Jotham Suez, Tal Korem, David Zeevi et al., 'Artificial sweeteners induce glucose intolerance by altering the gut microbiota', *Nature: International Weekly Journal of Science* 514 (2014): 186.

8. Rejuvenate

1. Justin Sonnenberg and Erica Sonnenberg, *The Good Gut* (London: Penguin Press, 2015), 112.
2. Antonio Jimenez-Escrig, Eva Gomez-Ordonez et al., 'Antioxidant and prebiotic effects of dietary fiber co-travellers from sugar Kombu in healthy rats', *Journal of Applied Psychology* 25 (2013).
3. Sonnenberg and Sonnenburg, *The Good Gut*, 91.
4. Sonnenberg and Sonnenberg, *The Good Gut*, 85.

9. Top It Up

1. Shonali Sabherwal, *The Beauty Diet* (New Delhi: Random House, 2012).

10. Oxygenate

1. Paul Pitchford, *Healing with Whole Foods,* (Berkeley: North Atlantic Books, 1993), 78.
2.   Dr Kazuhiko Asai, *Miracle Cure: Organic Germanium,* (Self-published, 1980).
3. Gerard E. Mullin, MD, *The Gut Balance Revolution* (Emmaus, PA: Rodale Books, 2015), location 5059.
4. Mullin, *The Gut Balance Revolution,* 5162.